YOUR HEALTH IN YOUR HANDS

Dr Ledermann is trained in general and psychological medicine, as well as in natural methods of healing. He is a well-qualified and experienced counsellor of those who enjoy contemporary life, but are threatened by its harmful consequences. He has been a consultant physician at the Royal London Homeopathic Hospital, and is a Fellow of the Royal College of Psychiatrists.

Your Health in Your Hands
A case for
natural medicine

E.K. Ledermann

MD FFHom FRCPsych

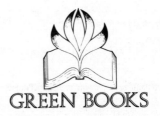

GREEN BOOKS

To the memory of
MY MOTHER

First published in 1989 by
Green Books
Ford House, Hartland
Bideford, Devon   EX39 6EE

Typeset by M R Reprographics
42 High Street, Chard
Somerset   TA20 1Q

Printed by Hartnoll
Victoria Square, Bodmin, Cornwall

Your Health in Your Hands
is printed on recycled paper

British Library Cataloguing in Publication Data

Ledermann E.K. (Erich Kurt), *1908-*
Your Health in Your Hands: A case for natural medicine.
1. Medicine. Naturopathy
I. Title II. Ledermann, E.K. (Erich Kurt),
1908- Good health through natural therapy
615.5'35

ISBN 1-870098-12-9

Contents

Preface

The phrase 'your health is in your own hands', sets the theme: people are responsible for their health, and they should not pass on this responsibility to others. This is an antidote to the prevalent idea that we are subject to forces over which we have no control. Doctors, trained in the science of medicine, are accepted as bearers of responsibility for the health of the lay population. I am not denying that medical science and their representatives are important, but people are not just the material which is investigated and treated by medical scientists. People are individuals and are unique; they have the freedom to decide how they wish to live.

A person's life style is a major factor in that person's health or illness. Doctors enlighten the public with regard to matters of health, including avoiding the dangers of smoking and of eating the wrong foods. This is called health education and through this people are granted the freedom to choose.

Science does not deal with individuals, it deals with whole classes of phenomena. In medicine it deals with diseases and individual people are said to be bearers of these. The scientific classification is fragmentary, it isolates phenomena. Patients are diagnosed as sufferers from pneumonia, appendicitis or depression and specific treatments are prescribed: penicillin, an operation, an anti-depressant drug. None of this is wrong in itself, but this approach makes no allowance for the individual personality's role in bringing about the state of ill health and in enduring it and making the effort to correct it.

So many people feel ill without suffering from some major illness which doctors can diagnose and treat with their specific powerful measures. They attend chemists and buy all sorts of tonics and mixtures some of which doctors would consider to be 'placebos', inert substances, just to please people. But these agents are not harmless. They frequently only relieve symptoms of ill health, of tiredness, indigestion, aches and pains which are calling for a change in life style, for a responsible attitude towards health which will eliminate the state of reduced health which has been brought about by faulty living.

An Alternative Natural Medicine is the title of the second part of this book. This form of medicine represents an alternative to analytical scientific medicine. Natural medicine is holistic and holism stands for the innate healing powers on which health and recovery from illness depend. Our modern technological age with its artificiality offends against the workings of the integrative forces of nature, manifest in the ecology, the natural surroundings. This interference is stressed as an important factor in the production of ill health. A natural medicine calls on people to show responsibility and to make an effort to redress the disturbed balance.

The scope of the natural alternative, a health obligation, is a major subject of the text, which details how to harness the healing forces of nature. The limitations of this approach are not denied and scientific medicine is presented as a necessary stand-by. In this way, I hope to avoid dogmatism.

Dr E.K. Ledermann
London, April 1988

The book contains applications of natural therapy, published as a hardback by the author in 1976 under the title *Good Health Through Natural Therapy,* and published as a paperback in 1978. In the present volume natural therapy is presented in the context of a holistic and ecological approach to medicine.

Acknowledgements
I should like to thank Ian K. Hutchinson, DC.(USA) and Carina A. Petter, DO, MRO for their assistance in formulating the sections on chiropractic and osteopathy respectively.

Introduction

Nature's balance

As a biological organism your life is in the hands of nature. But your life is threatened by the ecological crisis, by the disharmony and imbalance within the natural environment. This crisis is the result of an attitude which has led to an exploitation of biological resources by technological science. As one modern writer has put it, 'the fullest exploitation of nature involves its eventual destruction'.[1] It is the aim of this book to criticize this attitude and to focus on a different one that avoids such danger.

The difference between the two approaches consists in an emphasis on analysis and fragmentation which is characteristic of science and on wholeness which is the safeguard against the results of scientific fragmentation. The significance of the two approaches for your health will be shown in the various sections of the book. A holistic approach will be basic. It cannot claim to convey knowledge which is based on the discovery of mechanisms as in a machine; it rests on a conviction that life is ultimately inscrutable and, in Albert Schweitzer's words, demands reverence.

When Schweitzer started his hospital in the pristine, natural surroundings of equatorial Africa, there was harmony in the forest, a balance of animal and plant life. But the natives suffered from severe illnesses which required his scientific medical treatment. Therefore, ecological balance in nature may be accompanied by imbalance in the health of the people living in the area.

No unprejudiced person can deny that medical science is necessary for people. It has brought about the elimination of epidemics of cholera, typhus, and the black death which used to decimate the populations of Europe. It has still to conquer water-borne diseases, malaria and other infections which cause havoc in Asia and Africa. Such advances in health can only be achieved by controlling harmful agents in the environment.

The soil

This destruction of harmful organisms in the environment has been applied to plant life in the form of *insecticides* and *pesticides* and has led to an imbalance in the natural environment. As toxic substances they destroy the balance between pests and the other creatures which prey on them. They have delayed consequences which cannot be foreseen. Even if they are used correctly and not in excess, they may be spread by the wind and upset soil and plant ecology.

> Pesticides are only the most notorious of a vast multitude of man-made compounds which by now ⟦1972⟧ number at least half a million, with new ones arriving at a rate of 500 a year. Since it is costly to test the potential toxicity of new substances, the chances of a thorough investigation, at the moment, are not high. Man's water supplies are constantly being contaminated with substances the long-term effects of which are largely unknown.[2]

The soil is a living structure which consists of bacteria, fungi, algae, protozoa and other microscopic animals. They convert dead organic matter into its constituents and thus recycle it so that it becomes available for life again. The blue-green algae in particular inhabit the top millimetre or so of the soil, fixing nitrogen from the atmosphere and thus promoting the yield of this vital substance in a natural way. In fact they contribute between one-quarter and one-third of the available nitrogen for crops. This mass of organisms is critical to the basic biological process.

If human and animal excreta were put back into the soil, the soil would not be depleted. Agro-industrial science, however, depends on artificial chemical fertilizers and these make the soil vulnerable. In Holland, for instance, one researcher has found over-treated soil which has been made sterile with chemicals.[3] A further serious hazard to the soil comes from sludge containing industrial waste. Toxic metals, especially lead, cadmium, nickel and arsenic, and residues from chemical pesticides persist in the soil and are concentrated in plants. The dangerous effect of these toxic substances on animals and men has been overlooked.[4]

One chemical fertilizer, nitrate, used extensively in high-technology farming, is particularly dangerous. The danger consists in its conversion into nitrite which is toxic to people and animals. Babies are particularly sensitive to nitrite which enters drinking water and may be stored in spinach. Many factors affect the conversion into nitrite - a particular strain of plant, certain cultivation methods whether under glass or in the open, the terrain, method of harvesting, time of the year, temperature, as well as the type of storage of the vegetables before they are sold. For instance, the highest readings were recorded in *spring* cabbage grown in the United Kingdom.[5]

A simple alternative method available to gardeners is *composting;* this gives humus, a mixture of animal and vegetable residues produced through the agencies of micro-organisms. Through this process the natural cycle of life takes place without any harmful side-effects, the inorganic elements passing into organic ones. Composting can be carried out in different ways. The humus includes a base such as earth, wood-ash, chalk, sea-sand or a mixture of these. The base reduces the acidity. Water and air are also essential. Intense fermentation sets in which causes a rise in temperature, and fungi and bacteria act to break down the material. It was claimed by one expert, Sir Albert Howard,[6] that humus confers on plants resistance to disease which cannot be obtained by chemical artificial fertilizers.

Air and water
Obviously damage to the soil and indirectly to human health can be caused by pollution of the air and of the water which enters the soil. Acid rain is an example of such damage. It is partly caused by car fumes containing nitrogen oxides, and partly by emissions from power stations containing toxic sulphur dioxide. Acid rain has caused widespread environmental damage particularly in Scandinavia, where lakes have been rendered almost lifeless, and in Scotland where it has damaged lakes and the soil. It is responsible for the destruction of millions of trees in many countries, and has affected agricultural crops, buildings, wildlife and human health.

Some of the damage to people's health is due to acid rain leaching aluminium from the soil, from which it passes into human food mainly through water pollution.

Recent studies in Norway have shown a very close correlation between the incidence of Alzheimer's disease, a particularly unpleasant form of senile dementia, and levels of aluminium in the water. A further correlation is found between the high aluminium levels, and the areas of highest acid rain in Norway.[7]

Ozone, also a result of pollution by cars, damages trees and human health.[8] Like nitrogen oxides and sulphur dioxide ozone can travel for up to 2,000 kilometres, and during the hot summer months, the ideal conditions for its formation, its pollution clouds cover hundreds of miles. Ozone is formed by the combination of nitrogen oxide and hydrocarbons.

Lead, derived from petrol and released from vehicle exhausts, causes blood levels which are dangerous to health, especially the health of children, leading to restricted mental development.[9]

Carbon monoxide is another pollutant from car exhausts. It reduces the oxygen-carrying ability of red blood cells and aggravates chronic respiratory and cardiac disorders in susceptible people. 'In London, peak values can reach more than seven times the World Health Organisation recommended levels for long periods.'[10]

Hydrocarbon emissions from vehicles fuelled by petrol and diesel adhere to smoke particles and are inhaled. Like cigarette smoke they are a major cause of lung cancer, especially in urban areas.[11] This source could account for some 3,000 extra deaths per annum in the United Kingdom.[12] Diesel fuel is much more likely to induce disease than other fuel, yet legislation does not provide any safeguard against its abuse.

Carbon dioxide and other trace gases allow dangerous solar radiation to penetrate the earth's protective ozone layer, a barrier against harmful ultraviolet light from the sun. They originate from air-conditioning units and refrigerants, which have a massive market in the United States and Japan.[13]

Aerial spraying of pesticides - natural and manufactured ecology
Pesticides, we saw, harm the life of the soil and plant ecology. They are also a danger to human health. When inhaled they can cause vomiting and breathlessness; exposure to spraying can result in inflammation of the eyes; and headaches and skin troubles can result from contact with the skin. But reports of effects also include cases of impotence, the birth of a deformed baby, and deaths of young babies. Severe allergies and food intolerance can follow exposure to spraying. Although many farmers consider pesticides to be essential, their own health and that of their farm workers may be affected. 'With less pesticides there would be less damage to the environment, lower residues in food and drinking water, and a chance for wildlife to re-establish itself in the farmed countryside.'[14]

One author contrasts 'natural ecology' with 'a manufactured human ecology', brought about by the 'technological age man' who is unable to 'return to an isolated unit subsisting within natural ecology', as his civilization has led to often enormously large communities, vast urban conglomerations which are far removed from nature.[15] The same author insists that 'man must now develop new attitudes towards achieving a civilization which balances the two ecologies, natural and man-made'.[16]

The responsibility for achieving this balance and for developing this new attitude lies with those in authority, the governments which plan man-made ecology. Individual people can join pressure groups to try to influence the authorities. In their own lives people can try to protect themselves against the worst excesses of the ecological crisis. The growth of health-food shops, selling food unadulterated by chemicals, wholemeal instead of white bread, meat which does not contain the hormones or antibiotics so often fed to farm animals, is an indication of the public's determination to lead a more natural life. Health-food shops buy their goods from organic farmers who avoid the use of chemical fertilizers, pesticides and insecticides, thus achieving a holistic balance on their land. Their products, although more expensive than those of ordinary farmers, are in great demand which makes their efforts financially viable. Even more is to be gained if a farmer restores the soil, exhausted by exploitation over many years, to health and productivity. This holistic approach is valid for the promotion of human health. It is distinguished from the scientific-analytical approach of conventional medical science. The claims of the two schools of thought must now be examined.

Part One
Scientific and holistic medicine of the body

Chapter 1

Whom can you trust with your health?

As a lay person you may well be confused when you hear claims and counterclaims about medicine. The media have given wide coverage to 'unorthodox' practices; acupuncture, homoeopathy, osteopathy and chiropractic are praised for their efficacy although they do not form part of the official medical curriculum. Lay practitioners are not the only ones to employ these methods. The medical profession has founded a Holistic Association both in this country and in America. The *British Medical Journal,* the official publication of the British Medical Association, has admitted that the number of lay practitioners in 1981 in the United Kingdom was 27,800, compared with 29,800 general medical practitioners in 1982! In the same article a Scottish doctor, training to be a general practitioner, revealed that out of eighty-six colleagues seventy were not satisfied that their training had given them sufficient knowledge for their work. They therefore turned to alternative methods.[1] In *'Medicine out of Control: the Anatomy of a Malignant Technology'* an Australian doctor claims that modern medicine has been 'oversold', that the public has been misled by the claims that 'modern medicine is making great strides in its war against disease'.[2] He justifies this by stating that 'since the early 1900s there has not been a substantial further decline in adult mortality, particularly in males' and he gives as the reason, that 'the ''degenerative'' diseases of ''civilization'' (such as coronary heart disease) have cancelled out all gains from the further decline of infection'.[3] He denies that modern drugs, antibiotics and vaccines have conquered infectious diseases, that 'biomedical technology' can claim such a success. The reduction of these illnesses, he proves, is due to improved nutrition, sanitation, clean water supply, personal hygiene, better housing and a general improvement of social conditions. He warns readers not to be optimistic with regard to cancer where the 'situation has changed little in the last 50 years, and even less in the last 20', in spite of the use of very advanced technology.[4] Social and environmental factors play a major role in the incidence of viral diseases affecting lungs and bowels, in high blood pressure, diabetes and heart diseases. He also warns his readers of the danger of contracting diseases while under treatment in a hospital and of suffering damage through 'diagnostic technology'. These strident criticisms are not without confirmation from colleagues. A medical authority, a Nobel Prize winner, expressed his pessimism with regard to progress in medicine by saying that in his opinion modern research in the medical sciences offered hardly any hope for prevention of disease nor for improvement of health.[5]

A recent survey of the health of people in Great Britain and the USA has confirmed an unsatisfactory state of affairs. It points out that in spite of all the technological advances in scientific medicine, people in Britain and in America are in poor health. Since the turn of the century there has been little decline in cancer, arthritis, diseases of the heart and blood vessels, of the lungs, especially bronchitis and emphysema, of diabetes and depression. Cancer and mental illnesses are 'steadily increasing'. For Britain the incidence of cancer is 'some 200,000 cases every year'. For America the forecast is that 'one in every three Americans will get cancer before he turns 74'. Thirty-five million Americans suffer from high blood pressure 'which is a central cause of 1 ¼ million heart attacks and 500,000 strokes every year. Here in Britain more than 150,000 people die each year from the same conditions.' The writer of this article correctly points out that these diseases are 'the result of how we live, our nutrition, the way we cope with stress, how much physical activity we get and what kind of environmental pollution-radiation, airborne chemicals in our food we have to cope with'. The writer reminds the reader that these facts are known to 'even the most orthodox physician', and she calls for 'a more ecological approach to health' and for a reform in our eating 'which deviates too far from what our bodies have been genetically programmed over many thousands of years to expect'. Hence, she argues, we suffer from 'progressive malnutrition on a cellular level which in turn depresses the functioning of the body's immune system and eventually generates illness'.[6]

The question must be asked: why do scientifically trained doctors, in possession of the relevant knowledge, not prevent such diseases by applying their knowledge? The answer is that they are hampered by a traditional approach characterized by an emphasis on analysis and fragmentation, and which considers people to be objects of science and not free to act responsibly. People rely on the 'experts' to prevent or cure diseases and are not committed to the acceptance of a responsibility for their own health. The population is misled by the rosy forecasts made by medical science. The science of heredity and the prospects it holds out are one example of this. Heredity plays a major role in disease. The scientist locates the hereditary factor in the genes and modern medical science is experimenting with correcting faults in genes with 'genetic engineering'. But the editor of the *New Scientist* considers that 'the conditions amenable to this approach form a distinct and rare group. They are almost eclipsed by diseases for which this strategy would be irrelevant, unnecessary and ineffective.' This branch of science is called molecular medicine. Ageing is a hereditary phenomenon, but 'the notion that molecular medicine could be harnessed to thwart the natural course of ageing is a cruel mirage'.[7]

If you cannot trust promises of successful treatment and of further progress by medical science, does it follow that you should put your trust in those who offer an alternative? What do these practitioners, lay or medical, provide that the establishment does not? The two leading medical journals in this country, the *British Medical Journal* and the *Lancet*, and a well-known American medical journal, the *New England Journal of Medicine*, staunchly defend medical science and issue strong warnings against trust in an alternative approach.[8]

Different points of view
In order to understand and to resolve the conflict between those who claim a monopoly for medical science and those who offer an alternative we must clarify and examine further the foundations on which claims and counterclaims are based. You may wish to know which side has better results, cures more patients. But such a question is misleading. People brought up in our scientific age expect to be cured of a *disease*, for that is the way doctors tend to think. There are, however, no diseases, only sick people. Medical science distinguishes between physical and mental disease, each the province of a different department of medicine. But a person is a unity of body, mind and spirit, a unique individual and not just a 'case' of pneumonia or appendicitis or anxiety neurosis. After a specific diagnosis has been made, specific therapy for the disease is instituted. The results of such treatments are assessed critically. Medical scientists are rightly critical and sceptical. If

somebody quotes the history of a person who was 'cured' after conventional medical treatment had failed, the scientist is not convinced. The evidence is 'anecdotal', it is not proof, for the patient may have recovered in any case. What is required is statistical proof. To gain this, a large number of patients, suffering from the same disease to a comparable degree of severity, are treated with the curative agent in question. The results are compared with those from an equal number of people, suffering from the same condition and affected in the same way, but who have been treated with a dummy (placebo). Neither the patients nor those who gather the results must know whether a particular case has received the agent or has acted as a control. Only if the results obtained from the active agent are statistically better than those obtained with the placebo, can the agent be considered to be effective. The writer of the article in the *British Medical Journal,* referred to above, states that any doctor who treats a few patients (and he *can* only treat a few to start with) with an alternative method is acting in a way which is 'scientifically and ethically unacceptable'. Any treatment must first have been 'validated by a clinical trial' (i.e. by using the control method).[9]

The practitioner who considers himself to be concerned with the whole individual patient is a 'holist'. He may refuse to accept the scientific point of view on which the clinical control trial is based. If he practises holistic medicine, does he follow a medicine which is 'a pablum of common sense and nonsense offered by cranks and quacks and failed pedants who share an attachment to magic and an animosity toward reason', as the American authors in their journal maintain? He may well object to the view that he has 'joined forces with cranks and quacks, magicians and madmen'.[10] The *Lancet* simply states categorically 'Alternative medicine is no alternative'[11], but one reader strongly objected to this 'ignorant unsigned editorial full of innuendo' and to its 'aunt-Sally title' and insisted that there should be an end to this type of article.[12] He was convinced that osteopathy, for example, should be combined with scientific medicine. He thus agreed with those young doctors who seek knowledge, not supplied by their training, as necessary additions to their work. Many doctors send their patients to non-medical practitioners such as osteopaths without awaiting the results of a 'scientific' trial of osteopathy.

You might ask whether you can avoid having to make a choice between alternatives and simply have osteopathic treatment incorporated within your conventional medical therapy. But the Principal and Clinic Director of the European School of Osteopathy disagrees with such a compromise. He claims that 'osteopathy is a complete system of medicine' and not just 'a technique that can become part of other, complementary therapies. It exists in its own right, independent.' [13] You can expect to receive the same sort of answer with regard to homoeopathy and acupuncture.

Thus these unconventional methods do not necessarily represent alternatives to a patient, but they do represent alternative forms of thought. Before we can try to formulate how their effectiveness can be tested, we must first clarify the principles on which conventional medical science is based and which will, we hope, enlighten us with regard to the nature of the clinical trial. We will also have to grasp the principles underlying holistic medicine.

Chapter 2

Science in relation to your body

Mechanistic science

We have already gained some insight into the way in which medical scientists understand the human organism. By identifying individual diseases and by isolating the factor which is responsible for a recovery from a particular disease, the scientist uses the method of *analysis*. This means that the complexity of the whole is understood in terms of its parts. In the diagnosis the patient becomes the bearer of a particular abnormality which may be in one of his parts (organs), or may be due to the presence of some abnormal invading agent. Doctors thus speak of bronchial asthma if the airways in the lungs have become constricted and of septicaemia if the blood stream has been infected with some harmful germ. As the diagnosis is specific-analytical, so is the appropriate treatment: in the first case a drug is administered which dilates the bronchial tubes, in the second case an antibiotic is given which is active against the particular infection. If a vital substance such as the thyroid hormone is missing, the deficiency is made good by the prescription of this hormone. High blood pressure is lowered by reducing the tension in the wall of the arteries by certain drugs which may also reduce the blood volume through stimulating the kidneys to excrete more urine. Other drugs benefit these patients by reducing the output of blood by the heart. The pharmacologist and the physiologist who investigate these individual processes and their relationships discover the *mechanisms* which are isolated within the complexity of the living organism. The surgeon who removes diseased appendices or gall-bladders or who transplants kidneys or hearts or who dilates the narrowed lower end of the oesophagus employs another form of mechanistic treatment.

The English philosopher R.G. Collingwood has clarified the principle and has also opened our eyes to the restrictive and potentially harmful effects of the mechanistic approach. He identified mechanism as a hallmark of science. 'Mechanism', he explained, 'implies the ignoring of the omnipresent individuality of the real ⟦ in the case of medicine of a real person, the individual patient⟧ and the imposition upon it of an abstract law which determines every case indifferently from the outside', the 'law' being the analytical medical approach.[1] The patient's real individuality may affirm itself by the way in which it responds with more or less serious 'side-effects' to the treatment. The result is called 'iatrogenic' (physician-caused) disease. Such adverse reactions to drugs amount to 10-20 per cent in hospital in-patients and to lengthening of hospital stay because of their severity in 2-10 per cent of patients who are suffering from an acute illness.[2] A medical authority comments on the dangerous consequences which follow the pharmacological application of mechanistic medicine by admitting that 'our powers over nature in applied pharmacology have extended so far that nature seems to have become retaliatory and is exacting a heavy retribution'.[3] To the dangers from prescribed drugs must be added the danger from sophisticated diagnostic procedures and diagnostic technology.[4] These hazards contribute greatly to a loss of faith in medical science and to the turning to alternative forms of treatment. The flaw in mechanistic medical thinking must be exposed further by demonstrating the fundamental difference between the living organism and the lifeless machine.

Your body is not a machine

Technological processing is carried out by machines which are whole structures, analysable into their component parts. Their functions are fully explained by the relationships between the parts which were earlier defined as the mechanistic explanation of science.

The medical scientist is tied to the mechanistic approach. This bond accounts for his successes which, we saw, consist in specific treatments, based on specific diagnosis. It also accounts for the failure to conquer cancer and degenerative diseases, especially those affecting the blood vessels in the heart and brain, which lead to heart attacks and to strokes.

A British physiologist has shown conclusively that the body is fundamentally different from a machine. He made the difference clear by distinguishing between two types of relationship which prevail between the parts of a whole. In the machine, the relationship between the parts is 'external' which means that their properties are not affected when they are removed from the machine-whole. Because of this externality, the repair of a faulty machine is carried out by first identifying which part is faulty and then by correcting the fault or by replacing the part.

The medical scientist acts like the mechanic. His diagnosis consists in discovering the specific 'disease' and the treatment is a surgical or medical correction. The failures of scientific medicine stem from the fact that in a living whole the parts are 'internally' related which means that 'the properties of a part are different when it is in its place in the organic hierarchy from what they are when it is removed from it'.[5]

Machines and living bodies both have hierarchical features. Both operate with feedbacks although the two feedbacks are different and glandular biological structures have nothing in common with the material structures of which machines are composed. Can the body then not be considered in analogous fashion to a machine? Analogous stands as different from identical.

Energy is required for the performance of glandular activity, for the maintenance of your body temperature, for muscular movements in your body including the movement of your heart muscle, and for your breathing. This energy is derived from the food which you consume. It is measured in heat units or calories. These are provided by protein, carbohydrate and fat, and tables of the calorific values of the different foods which contain these nutrients are often given. Further tables state the energy requirements of people of different ages, sexes, occupations and heights. Values are given for all the usual foods which include, for example, white bread, wholemeal bread, polished and unpolished rice, chocolate, and alcohol in different forms. Thus the machine scientist ignores the health aspect when calculating energy requirements. In fact, his science is not really accurate. While the fuel consumption, say, of a certain type of motor car can be correctly calculated (all cars of this make have the same consumption), people even if scientifically comparable can vary in their requirements by 20 per cent. Thus one man of a certain height and a certain age, resting in bed, might need 2,200 calories per day, while a man of the same height and age, also resting in bed, might balance his needs with an intake of 1,800 calories. Emotional factors also affect your needs. The energy concept makes no allowance for the benefit derived from fasting or from a reduced intake of food which, we shall see, may be of great therapeutic value to your health. During such periods people use up reserves stored in their bodies and different people respond quite differently to the temporary reduction of energy supply.

Your body deals with the food you eat in a way which is completely different from the way in which a machine functions. Although the chewing and digestive processes can be compared with mechanical and chemical processes, the breakdown of nutrients forms a common pool from which all the cells of the body select material for growth - in the case of children - and for reconstruction throughout life. The cells are not fixed units like the bricks of which a house is built. Every cell continuously renews its composition, rebuilding itself, giving up elements into the pool and selecting elements from it. No machine functions in this way.

Many people in our society are overweight. If you should suffer from obesity, you may discover that eating less will not necessarily make you slim. You may be gaining weight more readily than others who eat more than you do. The medical scientist explains your dilemma by suggesting that you conserve energy more than thin people do and that your fat tissue is different from that of those who are not fat. Thus there is no balance of energy intake and output as one finds in a machine.

Further evidence for the organic, non-mechanistic activity of the body can be derived from the development of the embryo which is not explained by the mechanistic process of the splitting of the hereditary substances.

Thus the mechanistic principle cannot account for organic life, only a non-mechanistic, holistic principle can do justice to the phenomena of life including the functioning of your body.

Chapter 3

Wholeness in relation to your body

The idea of wholeness

Your body as a manifestation of nature's creative power functions as a whole. The need to consider your body holistically is deduced from the fact that all the parts are related to each other 'internally'. The destructive effects of food technology on the life within the soil and the dangers which follow and threaten your health all call for a clear understanding of the holistic principle in relation to your body.

In order to account for the wholeness of a living thing, plant or animal or human being understood biologically, we employ the *idea of purpose.* We can understand the function of the heart only by understanding its purpose, that of pumping blood into the arteries. The purpose of the kidneys for the maintenance of the body is understood as the elimination of certain toxic material, the lungs fulfil the purpose of providing the whole body with oxygen and of getting rid of carbon dioxide.

Heart, kidneys, lungs and all the other parts, however, in fact *have* no purpose. Kant reminded us that by using the term 'purpose' we introduce a subjective human element into biology. Our minds have purposes. Therefore we judge the living body 'on an analogy with our own causality'.[1] Kant called this judgement regulative or heuristic. By making it, we reflect on the inner relationship which guarantees the integration of all the parts. Such reflection enables us to discover what role is played by the various parts in the maintenance of the whole. But, Kant insisted, we must not pretend that we explain the constitution of the living thing by our judgement which is based on analogy. Living things are thus *inscrutable.* In order to make sense of them, we have to look at them *as if* they had been designed, as if they expressed an end or telos. We are thus obliged to use a teleological judgement. Understanding life in that way means that we project the idea of a whole-making life force on biological phenomena to account for growth, integration and healing.

Health: wholeness of your body

Health depends on holistic growth and integration. But health is not a subject for medical science, for this science, as we saw, is concerned with fragmentation. The National Health Service in Great Britain is really a National Disease Service.

While scientists investigate only particular aspects, for instance the processes which take place when we breathe, they can and ought to relate each particular aspect of life to the life of the whole body. They locate a breathing centre in the brain and they may describe it 'as a computer which receives information' from various parts of the body 'to calculate the demand for ventilation'.[2] The term 'computer' is misleading if you ignore the fact that it is used only in an analogous way, comparing what happens in a living organism with what happens in a machine, constructed and programmed by the human mind. Our minds calculate, but cells in our brains which compose regulative centres do not do so. With our limited cognitive faculties we use words such as 'computer' to account for amazing co-operation of all the parts of our bodies.

As it is 'the purpose' of the lungs to provide the blood with oxygen and to remove carbon dioxide from it, respiration is co-ordinated with the circulatory system. As 'the purpose' of the kidneys is to excrete certain substances which are present in the blood, their functions are co-ordinated with the circulatory, and indirectly with the respiratory, systems.

While the co-ordination of these bodily functions occurs in an automatic way to some extent, the mind has a profound influence on it. You can train yourself to breathe more efficiently. You can become aware of how much your emotions affect your breathing: you hold your breath when you are frightened, you take a long breath when you are relieved of some anxiety. When you run, your breathing and your heart-rate are accelerated. Your kidneys are stimulated to excrete more urine when you are under emotional tension, which can be reduced through relaxation. Your skin is part of the integrative process of life: through its sweat glands it excretes water, salts and urea, all of which are also eliminated by your kidneys. As in the case of breathing, the activities of your skin are modified by the way in which you treat your body: the circulation and the secretions of the sweat glands can be stimulated by the application of heat and cold and by exercise. Your mind has a profound influence on the skin as well: blushing and blanching, for example, reflect embarrassment and fear.

The holistic significance of digestion and assimilation of the food you consume was stressed when we discussed food production and when we refuted the notion that your body is a machine. Not only is your state of nutrition an indication of your general overall health, but of great interest also is the state of balance between the types of micro-organisms in your bowel. Your health does to some extent depend on a healthy bowel 'flora' which is affected by the provision of fibre. Fibre, lacking in processed food, increases the bulk of the evacuation and the speed at which it passes through the bowel. It has been claimed that a high-fibre diet will protect against cancer of the bowel, one of the most common cancers in industrialized communities.[3] Dietary fibre has also been found to affect blood pressure: when volunteers decreased their dietary fibre, their blood pressure rose after four weeks on a fibre-deficient regime, whereas other volunteers who ate a diet rich in fibre showed a decrease in their blood pressure over the same period.[4] Medical scientists thus confirm that your bodily health depends on avoiding food which has been deprived of its wholeness. Medical scientists with their fragmentary and specific approach, we saw earlier, are not successful in preventing or curing what we called 'the degenerative diseases of civilization' which include heart disease and cancer. You do not rely on detailed scientific knowledge to prevent such ill-health. You can safeguard your health by wholesome living. While you cannot avoid all the stresses of life which endanger your health, you can avoid some.

Smoking

Smoking is 'the biggest avoidable menace to health in contemporary life in Britain'. It causes 'all told, ten times as many deaths as all cancers unrelated to smoking put together'. A cigarette smoker's chances of dying in middle age are twice those of a non-smoker. This situation is brought home by the statistics: two out of every five heavy smokers are likely to die before the age of 65, compared with only one out of every five non-smokers.[5] In Great Britain smoking is estimated to cause 100,000 deaths every year. The medical scientists have known since 1950 about 'the link between smoking and serious illness and death; [[during that time]] between one and a half and three million Britons must have died prematurely from [[this]], an avoidable cause'.[6] 'The United States Surgeon General estimates that 346,000 Americans die every year from smoking-related diseases'.[7] Medical scientists unravel the ways in which cigarette smoking damages the wholeness, the integrity of the body. They discover the damaging effects on lung structures and on blood vessels, including those which provide blood to the heart; they observe that smokers suffer from occupational allergies,[8] that the health of an unborn baby is harmed if the mother smokes during pregnancy. We can expect further scientific evidence, but such is unnecessary for those who are aware that cigarettes are unhealthy and should therefore not be smoked.

Alcohol
Alcoholism affects not only various parts of the body but also the mind via the brain. Alcohol abuse damages the stomach, the liver, the heart, the nerves, the pancreatic gland, and the unborn baby.

> As many as a million individuals in Britain suffer serious problems because of their drinking, and their problems inevitably affect the many millions who are their husbands, wives, children, parents, employers, and friends. Each year ... the deaths of 500 people under 25 (10% of all such deaths) result through drunkenness. In 1980 half a million admissions to general medical hospitals were linked with alcohol, while in 1979 almost 14,000 admissions to psychiatric hospitals were for 'alcoholism' and 'alcoholic psychosis'. Alcohol is also associated with 80% of deaths from fire, 65% of serious head injuries, half of all murders, 40% of road traffic accidents that include pedestrians, 35% of fatal accidents, a third of all domestic accidents, and 14% of drownings. A third of divorce petitions cite alcohol as a contributory factor, and in a third of all child abuse cases one parent drinks heavily. Eight million working days are lost every year through drink problems, and a conservative estimate by the Department of Health and Social Security puts the total annual cost for alcohol abuse through lost productivity, accidents, and the costs of treatment and social services at £650m for 1977-8 - the real figure for 1982 must be several times higher.[9]

People take to alcohol for different reasons. If you happen to be suffering from agoraphobia and social phobia, from fear of open spaces and fear of meeting people, a recent article in a psychiatric journal warns you not to use drink to overcome your fear:

> Sixty alcoholics (40 males) were assessed for agoraphobia and social phobia, and over half the sample were rated as having either or both of these disorders when last drinking .... The more severely phobic males were also found to be the most alcohol dependent .... All phobic alcoholics reported that alcohol had helped them to cope in feared situations, and almost all had deliberately used it for this purpose.[10]

The alcohol problem in the United States can be judged by the following report:

> More than half those questioned in a recent Harris poll in the United States reported that a member of their family or a close friend drank too much (*Journal of Public Health Policy 1985*:6:295-9). Alcohol, not drugs, should be seen as the number one health problem in young people: it is an important factor in child abuse and family break ups, while alcohol related traffic accidents are the main cause of death in the under 25s.[11]

Alcohol dependence is common not only in young people. A recent investigation has found that 13 per cent of people aged 60 to 95 years, men and women, married and single, in social class III, living in Newcastle upon Tyne 'drank enough to put them at risk from alcoholic liver disease ... 〚 and 〛 a similar study of the elderly in New York reported 20% of men and 2% of women to be heavy drinkers.'[12]

Tea and coffee

The dangers of being dependent on smoking and on drinking are well-known, but the dangers of a dependence on tea and coffee, although far less serious, are less well-known. 'A heavy user may be defined as one who takes more than 5 cups of coffee (100-150 mg. caffeine per cup) and 12 cups of tea (40 mg. caffeine per cup) per day.'[13] Many people in Great Britain and especially in Ireland are dependent on tea and/or coffee. They are often not aware of the harmful effects: headache, irritability, jitteriness, tension and anxiety. If they suffer from a duodenal or stomach ulcer, tea and coffee make the complaint worse. People also suffer from allergies to tea and coffee which can take many different forms. Because tea contains tannin, it can interfere with absorption of iron from food and can thus contribute to anaemia.[14] Other symptoms include palpitations and sleep disturbance. When people give up these beverages, they suffer from withdrawal effects, especially headaches, irritability, inability to work effectively, lethargy and restlessness, nausea and drowsiness. 'Not surprisingly, caffeine withdrawal headaches respond to caffeine but tend to recur the next day.'[15] In a recent article further important dangers of caffeine consumption in high quantities were reported: anxiety and depression in college students, panic attacks, high blood pressure and heart failure with rapid heart-rate and palpitations, sleeplessness, diminution of intellectual power, and abnormal behaviour. 'A growing number of authorities have voiced their alarm and recommended moderation in the use of the drug.' It is recognized that 'there is no reason to assume that all individuals will be equally responsive to caffeine intake and/or withdrawal'.[16] This qualification by the scientists does not affect the holists' judgement that the drug caffeine is harmful as it interferes with the natural functioning of the organism, even if the damage is apparent only in some people.

Further recent information about even a moderate consumption of caffeine concerns the danger in pregnancy: it substantially increases the chance of spontaneous miscarriages in the later months of pregnancy.[17]

Health: your responsibility

Medical scientists keep you informed of the outcomes of their research. You are told of the dangers to your health from drinking excessive amounts of tea and coffee, of the dangers of even small amounts if you are allergic to caffeine. You are warned against becoming dependent on alcohol, and about the dire consequences of smoking. An editorial in the *British Medical Journal* accuses the government of having done 'virtually nothing' to curb cigarette smoking. The writer entitles his paper 'The avoidable holocaust' with a subtitle 'Past irresponsibility'. He insists first that 'the risks [[of smoking]] must be continually brought to the public's attention', that more research is needed 'into giving up smoking'. Secondly, the author of the paper cites as proof of the power of the 'addictive habit' that 'a fifth of doctors still smoke' although they are 'fully cognisant of all the risks'. Smokers 'need sympathetic help to stop and stay abstinent.' Thirdly, the government should 'impose swingeing taxes on cigarettes and lighten those on safer forms of nicotine, such as pipes, cigars, and snuff, as well as removing tobacco altogether from the cost index'. The next demand is: 'our Government needs to express society's disapproval of the habit' by enforcing non-smoking regulations in public places, banning advertising and avoiding sponsorship by tobacco companies. These demands are put forward in order to save the lives and the health of British people. The final point made is that there should be an effort to avoid exporting cigarettes to the developing countries.[18]

It might be asked whether it is really the government's responsibility. The dangers of smoking have been made quite clear to everybody. They could be emphasized again, but ultimately people have to take responsibility for their health themselves.

Such obligation involves an awareness of the harmful consequences of certain habits and to resist such habituation. Important examples of such interference with wholeness of health are the harmful effects of seeking relief from tension by cigarettes, the harmful altered state of mind as a result of drinking alcohol, and the harmful stimulation experienced by consuming tea and coffee. All these social customs involve a particular person's health conduct. Further serious hazards are added because doctors are obliged by patients to offer relief from the stresses of life. Endless prescriptions for tranquillizers and sleeping pills are issued which often seriously interfere with bodily and mental health causing numerous side-effects. Doctors who resist the clamour for such relief appeal to their patients' courage to face their conflicts and deal with them, thus accepting responsibilities for their own lives.

A responsibility for a healthy life extends beyond avoiding all these artificialities. It involves efforts to avoid foods which have been tampered with, it involves attention to correct breathing, correct posture and to a balance between exercise and relaxation, all of which are the subjects of the second part of this book.

Many doctors pay lip service to these principles of healthy living. But their medical-scientific training is liable to sabotage the implementation of such principles. For medical scientists investigate individual processes and not wholeness. Before 1950 doctors had not discovered the mechanisms which prove smoking to be harmful, but from a holistic point of view such proof was unnecessary. With regard to tea and coffee a medical scientist has admitted that 'it is possible, on theoretical grounds, to make an imposing list of diseases which may be made worse by caffeine-containing drinks, but there is no conclusive evidence to warrant any general prohibitions'.[19] Of course, it is no question of a prohibition, only of advice to avoid any unnecessary damage to health.

The contraceptive pill, used by many millions of women, has been passed by medical scientists as safe for younger age-groups, but some members of the medical profession have taken a holistic view and have warned that the inhibition of ovulation by an action on a certain part of the brain which regulates the function of the ovaries is likely to have very serious dangers to health. Some have already been established, such as abdominal symptoms, damage to blood vessels and some emotional troubles. Others, more serious, are at present under investigation and no final conclusions have been reached. The risks of cancer of the womb and of the breast are being considered.

The holistic approach does not depend on detailed studies such as this: even before 1950 it had condemned smoking as detrimental to health without waiting for the scientific evidence; it is opposed to drinking coffee (especially in large amounts) and with regard to the contraceptive pill it shares the view of a leading member of the medical profession: 'I personally cannot believe that it is possible to interfere in a natural process for so long without something really serious happening.' [20]

The holistic approach relies on people's innate sense of responsibility for their health. It thus opposes the sale of convenience foods, boosted by the food industry irrespective of their risks to health, it also opposes the use of the contraceptive pill and advocates such harmless methods of birth control as the sheath and the diaphragm.

The holistic approach welcomes the ever increasing number of health shops which enable people to buy wholesome foods, accepting a responsibility for health as a personal commitment and not relying on government propaganda.

Chapter 4

Natural treatment: the test for holism

The attack upon holism by the medical establishment, expressed by leading medical journals, is directed against the claim that sickness can be treated in any other way but by medical science, by its specific approach. The writers in the American journal, quoted earlier, insist that there is no other model for treating the sick but the recognized scientific one, that holistic medicine lacks 'a recognized set of problems, shared standards for a solution of these and a critical exchange among its practitioners that is characteristic of the sciences'.[1] We must now meet this attack.

Our defence will be built on our refutation of the machine conception of the body and on its replacement by the idea of wholeness, the true guide to the understanding of organic nature.

There are many forms of holistic treatment, such as homoeopathy, acupuncture, osteopathy and chiropractic, but they cannot provide us with the arguments which we require. For the medical scientist would demand that we provide evidence that these measures are effective when compared with a dummy control. This evidence is not available at present.

We shall focus on what we have already established about the living body, on its integrative power, its 'internal' relationships. This power, we saw, is creative. It responds to changes in the conditions under which the organism functions and such responses are those of individual bodies and not of bodies in general. By outlining a medicine which has as its model the individual person, suffering from an illness affecting his or her body, we shall not accept the scientific classification according to specific diseases and their specific treatment. We shall not be concerned with the discovery of 'causal pathways of the body' which the American authors consider to be essential.[2]

Self-healing

The essential premise for our holistic natural treatment is our trust in the self-healing power of the sick organism. Therefore, if possible, any unnatural influence must be excluded so that self-healing can take place without interference. This means the sick person must try to avoid all the adverse factors which, we saw, make up such a common part of life in civilization: all the inessential additions to food, stimulants such as tea, coffee and alcohol. Drugs, unless essential for the preservation of life, are also excluded, as they have no place in the natural economy of organic life. In certain books on natural treatment the view that the body *inevitably* heals itself under appropriate conditions can lead to serious dogmatic statements. In a recent publication, the author Ross Trattler quotes with approval the 'truth', expounded by Lindlahr, an early pioneer of natural healing, that 'every acute disease is the result of a healing effort of nature'.[3]

This conception defines, as a 'major factor in almost all disease', an 'accumulation of toxic material within the body due to improper diet, poor circulation, poor elimination, and lack of demanding exercise'.[4] Suppressive drugs and vaccines are blamed for inhibiting the eliminative efforts of the body. They are thus condemned. Fever is welcomed as it speeds up the removal of toxins from the body, inflammation with its increased blood and lymph supply aids the natural defences, diarrhoea and vomiting are attempts of the body to rid itself of toxic substances. If the elimination of waste matter and poisons from the body is hindered, chronic disease results, due to the accumulation of waste materials and poisons, 'with consequent destruction of vital parts and organs'. The constructive and healing forces are 'no longer able to act against the disease conditions by acute corrective efforts (healing crisis)'.[5]

Trattler has modified this simplistic view and has admitted that drugs and surgery may be necessary in acute diseases. He still maintains that such conditions ought to have been prevented by a healthier life style, but, once the disease has occurred, he concedes that natural methods may not be sufficient to deal with it. For instance he holds that 'nearly any infection anywhere in the body can develop to the point that the use of antibiotics is a wise course of action', but he qualifies this point by saying: 'This, however, usually occurs only if the earliest signs of infection are ignored, or if the individual's vital energy and immunological resistance are depressed by poor diet or other factors [[so]] that the body is no longer capable of self-cure rapidly enough.'[6]

Thus fever and inflammation are no longer judged to be beneficial in all cases and drugs, employed to eliminate the infection and the accompanying fever, are no longer thought to be adding to the state of general illness. That concession is welcome, but his qualification is misleading: even if the earliest signs of infection are not ignored, antibiotics would be required if the infection is sufficiently *virulent*. In that case, 'the individual's vital energy and immunological resistance', even if not 'depressed by poor diet and other factors' would not save the case for natural treatment.

It is true that doctors prescribe antibiotics for many infections for which they are not needed and where they do harm through their side-effects. In such cases, the natural methods of dieting and water treatment (hydrotherapy) are effective and to be preferred to the use of drugs. The holistic treatments of homoeopathy, acupuncture, osteopathy and chiropractic represent important additions to the natural methods and their combination constitutes a powerful stimulation of the body's healing forces. The change in the patient's life style with the addition of the auxiliary methods brings about a profound change within the complicated holistic forces within the organism. This is evident in many ways which naturopaths are inclined to interpret as elimination of toxins and waste matter without being able to identify the chemical nature of such elements.

Correction of nutritional imbalance
Many practitioners of natural healing prescribe vast quantities of vitamins, minerals and other food supplements for their patients. They argue that the average diet does not provide these needed elements in sufficient quantities. They justify their practices with reference to the fact that the soil on which food has grown is frequently depleted, the principles of ecology having been neglected. They also claim that the methods of the food industry and the process of cooking cause such deficiencies.

These practitioners spoil their case when they admit that each person is unique in his or her biochemical make-up. In that case, supplements ought to be added if a lack of essential nutrients can be proved in a particular case. In fact, one advocate of these nutritional supplements, Ross Trattler,[7] does not classify patients according to their biochemical make-up but according to their diseases, thus using the classification of scientific medicine. Thus these supplements are prescribed in cases of osteo- and rheumatoid arthritis, bronchial asthma, whooping cough, dandruff, bed-wetting, epilepsy, in fact for any condition discussed in his book. The author admits that in some 'relatively rare conditions a genetic biochemical alteration has been recognized', a deficiency in enzymes which are essential for proper food assimilation. Of course, patients whose absorption of food from their stomach or intestines is deficient would qualify for supplements to their diet, but in hardly any disease dealt with in his book has this condition been fulfilled. This form of treatment has been named 'orthomolecular' which means 'right molecule'.

In one section of the book vitamin toxicity is discussed. It is admitted that vitamin A is 'highly toxic if taken to excess and toxicity can occur at supplemental level at or above 50,000 international units per day'. This warning is not heeded in the rest of the text, as only levels of vitamin A *above* 50,000 international units are said to require 'medical supervision'. In the case of bronchial asthma, the author prescribes for children Vitamin A: 10,000 international units two to four times a day without specifying the age of the child. For adults for the same condition, the amount is raised to 25,000 international units two to four times per day in acute cases, although the warning not to exceed 50,000 units per day without medical supervision is added.[8]

Other doubts arise when we are told that 'some naturopaths also employ glandular substances such as raw ovary concentrate, raw adrenal, raw pituitary, and others'. The reason for such a practice is that these substances are used 'to nourish the body's glandular system and strengthen it, and not as a traditional doctor might use a hormone extract, which naturopaths feel weakens the gland'.[9] We must ask how the naturopath knows which gland needs nourishing and strengthening? He is unlikely to have access to laboratories which would provide the answer. Doctors prescribe such hormones when a deficiency in a gland has been proved. They would strenuously deny that these necessary supplements have a weakening effect. The unnatural prescriptions of orthomolecular and glandular substances are not likely to correct nutritional imbalance, but rather intensify it.

Natural stimuli and your body's responses

When the responsibilities for your health were stressed, wholesome living, it was stated, consists in attention to natural food, to correct breathing, to a correct posture, to carrying out suitable exercises followed by periods of rest and relaxation. Exercise affects the rate of your heart as well as the depth of your breathing. The circulation within your skin and the excretion of sweat provide further opportunities for natural treatment, assisting the body in its recovery from illness. Life depends on *all* these activities and by suitable *modifications* of the conditions of life the natural therapist applies natural stimuli to which the patient's organism responds holistically. In the second part of the book an account of these treatments is given in some detail.

The modifications which affect the natural functions of the body are *graded* according to their intensity. The choice of a more or less drastic change will not primarily depend on your disease, as natural therapists do not use the classification according to diseases which forms the framework of scientific analytical medicine. The change will depend on how ill the patient is and on the responses that can be expected from various natural stimuli. *All* possible means of assisting the body in its recovery will be employed which is in contrast to scientific medicine which treats only the patient's diseases by specific interventions, whether by drugs or operations.

The practical guide to treatment surveys the different forms of diet which can evoke a healing response, it stresses the importance of correct breathing for health, examines the part played by the use of hot and cold water applied to the skin, and the importance of different forms of exercise. Each time, the treatment is matched to a particular organism's ability to *respond* and every healing response is interpreted as a manifestation of that creative mysterious power which maintains life.

Your mind's responses

Natural treatment is more than a whole-making treatment of your body. Although it is not a treatment for mental illness as such, it is a treatment of body, mind and spirit and does not suffer from the one-sidedness which characterizes the scientific approach which separates bodily (physical) medicine from psychological medicine. It is not forced into the straitjacket of specialization which restricts scientific medicine. The mind's response is evident in a number of ways.

Experience

You are aware of your body, especially when you are ill. In the second part of this book the emotional implications of natural treatment will be stressed. In the discussion of diet, the significance of hunger and the craving for certain foods will be considered. Your breathing, your posture, exercises and periods of relaxation will all be evaluated as important experiences, apart from their effects on your body.

Your recovery from bodily illness through natural treatment brings about a relief of pain and discomfort and a welcome revival of the senses of taste and smell. Your physical well-being is felt as a release from a malaise which in the case of chronic ill-health you had almost taken for granted. The relationship between your body and your mind is reciprocal. As your mental state improves, this improvement is reflected in your body. As you feel better, your digestion, your breathing, your heart and other organs benefit. You now enjoy carrying out exercises which before you felt unable to do. Your sleep may become more satisfactory with benefit to your bodily and mental state as a whole.

Preparedness
When suggesting the various changes in your life style with their accompanying emotional impact, your therapist has to assess not only the response of your body to such changes but also the response of your mind. For instance he will recommend a fast on water or on fruit juices only if you are prepared to face the experience of hunger and the feelings that go with it. If you are frightened and anxious, fasting will only harm you. As natural treatment consists in altering your habits, your general attitude will be decisive. The question of how conventional you are will be very important. Do you mind differing from other members of your family and from your friends when it comes to eating and drinking? Do you depend on their approval? Does your professional life oblige you to share in the taste of your colleagues and customers? The answers to these questions indicate whether you are prepared for a change in your habits.

Motivation
Whether people are prepared to respond to the suggestion that they change depends largely on their motivation, on how much they are determined to achieve the goal they have set themselves. If you accept responsibility for your health you will be prepared to forgo all unnecessary hazards such as the wrong foods, stimulants, smoking and excessive consumption of alcohol. You will also accept the responsibilities implied in treatment by natural means, the more or less drastic changes in your diet, the exercises, and the stimulation of the various functions of your body. Your motivation will depend on how convinced you are of the need to attain better health by adopting a healthier way of living. You will rely on your therapist to inform you to what extent it is necessary to modify your habits and for what period of time. The treatment is a challenge for you and your therapist appeals to

you to accept the challenge. The response to his appeal depends on your motivation, and on your determination to achieve better health through your own efforts, not relying on scientific medicine, and its drugs.

Your motivation will be strengthened if your therapist has set an example of wholesome living. Your self-confidence will grow as you feel that you are not an object of treatment but that you are a free agent in communication with your therapist. A sense of responsibility to health, stressed earlier, is essential to induce the right motivation.

Proofs of medical science and of natural treatment

We have investigated the principles on which natural treatment is based: the body is understood as an organic whole, its health depends on wholesome living, and in the event of illness health is restored by a suitable modification of your life style. Your mind is involved, as you, the subject, must take responsibility for your health. The success of natural treatment depends on your preparedness for the necessary changes in your habits and on your motivation. These are the results of our investigation and we can now decide whether natural treatment should prove its efficacy by submitting to the test demanded by the medical scientist. As you will remember, the scientist insists that the efficacy of any method should be proved by comparing its effects with those of a placebo or dummy. Neither the patient nor the therapist should know whether the alleged efficient agent or the placebo is being used.

This test is valid in the case of scientific medicine. It treats diseases, isolated phenomena, by a specific remedy which either influences the course of the disease favourably or fails to do so. If a placebo has the same effect as the alleged therapeutic agent, the agent is considered to be ineffective. The patient, the bearer of the disease, is an object of scientific enquiry into the efficiency of the alleged treatment. His whole and only responsibility is to take the prescribed remedy or placebo as directed by the medical scientist. In the scientific test the patient is lumped together with a sufficiently large number of people suffering to the same degree from the same complaint, to allow the medical scientist to evaluate statistically the result of the test. The patients in the group treated with the agent under consideration, and those in the control group given the placebo, must be comparable if the test is to be valid.

The test is inappropriate to natural treatment, for this approach views patients as individuals and unique people, each expected to cope with the challenge of their illness by altering those habits which have contributed to the illness. Natural treatment does not involve a single specific intervention such as a drug; it is a combination of various measures such as diet, water treatment, and exercises which stimulate the body's efforts to regain health. The response is not mechanistic and fragmentary but holistic, a response from the whole-making force of life.

Whether your body or your mind respond to your own illness, the validity of the natural holistic approach is not in question. For the stimuli which are applied to your body - a change of diet, cold or hot water applications to your skin, certain graded exercises - may have been too drastic or not drastic enough, but the principle according to which they were chosen remains valid: the self-healing tendency of the organism can be mobilized by changes in the conditions under which the person lives.

With regard to your mind's response, you may fail to summon the energy necessary for a healthier life, you may decide that smoking is too pleasurable to give it up, you are free to choose your personal life style. You may decide that strenuous unhealthy professional duties are more important than periods of rest and relaxation. In any case, you cannot disprove that people have a responsibility for their health as enunciated by natural therapy.

The role of scientific medicine

While natural treatment as a form of holistic therapy has passed the test, having established its validity, it has not passed the test as a therapeutic monopoly. It has not established itself as the *only* medical approach. Although nature's integrative healing power is a guide for the therapist, although he trusts it when suggesting to the patient certain modifications of his life style, he cannot trust this power absolutely. For nature is not always holistic and patients are liable to die from malformations and illnesses.

The natural therapist has to *assess* in every case of illness the likely healing response and whether in the course of treatment the expected response has in fact occurred. If the response is unlikely to occur or has not materialized, the therapist is under an obligation to use all the methods of mechanistic medical science.

For instance an attack of diarrhoea can be interpreted as a healing effort on the part of the patient's body to eliminate some toxic material. In that case the therapist would not interfere with nature's efforts. If, however, the patient has lost fluid and valuable salts to a dangerous extent, the therapist must take steps to replace these losses, for instance by the intravenous route. If the battle against invading germs promises to be successful with the employment of natural means, natural treatment is the correct approach. But if the infection is virulent and likely to overwhelm the body's natural defences, any available antibiotic must be used to assist in the struggle for recovery. The patient who acts as a subject, carrying out health-promoting changes in his life, accepting the therapist as an adviser with whom he communicates, becomes an object of medical science when his therapist treats him scientifically. He relies on the therapist's objective assessment of his condition throughout the treatment.

Apart from monitoring a patient's progress, assessing his needs for scientific medicine and employing scientific measures, the natural therapist may find the scientific approach useful when it confirms the value of his own methods. The natural therapist recommended a diet rich in fibre for certain bowel complaints when scientific medicine was warning against the use of roughage and insisting on bland diets. Now in the light of favourable results scientific medicine has accepted the value of a diet rich in fibre in these cases.

An even more fundamental change of attitude may come about as the result of certain reports published in the *New England Journal of Medicine*. The change relates to the interpretation of fever. To the natural therapist fever is a way in which the body rids itself of harmful substances and therefore is considered part of the self-healing tendency which is not interfered with unless it threatens the patient's life. The scientific view has been the very opposite. As the *New England Journal* reports, as recently as 1960, two eminent medical scientists 'in a comprehensive review could not adduce any conclusive evidence that fever was in itself of any benefit in the warfare between microbe and host'. Thus doctors, trained in scientific medicine, and the general public who follow their view, treat feverish patients with drugs such as aspirin to bring the temperature down (when specific infections are diagnosed, they use antibiotics). 'This view has been radically changed by [[the]] remarkable discovery': lizards' survival after being infected with a fever-producing agent is 'directly correlated with the elevated temperature'. Experiments with infected rabbits have yielded similar results.[10] A correspondent of the same journal asks in a letter: 'Will aspirin or acetaminophen treatment prolong the duration of colds or flu?'[11] In reply to the correspondent, the original author remarks:

> The practical deduction ... is that in infections that cannot be controlled by antibiotics, small elevations in body temperature (perhaps 102F to

104F) ⟦38.9°C to 40°C⟧ may be beneficial and are without evident harm to patients otherwise in good health and able to withstand the increased physiologic demands that fever imposes on the cardiorespiratory system.[12]

Thus the natural therapist finds his view of nature's whole-making tendency confirmed by a detailed investigation carried out by scientific medicine.

Conclusion

The answer to the question as to whom you can trust with your life and your health is, first of all, yourself, by taking the necessary steps to keep well. These are described by those practitioners who acknowledge the wholeness of nature. Should you fall ill, you should seek their guidance as to how to recover by modifications in your life style. These will be adjusted to your personal needs; they aim at a response from the healing power of nature, and from your own preparedness to make such changes. Your therapist may employ treatments in addition to natural therapy. These could include homoeopathy, acupuncture, osteopathy, chiropractic and massage. All of them rely on the whole-making power of nature and are thus allies to natural treatment.

If no recovery on holistic lines can be expected or has been achieved, the artificial measures of mechanistic, scientific medicine will have to be employed.

Part Two
An alternative natural medicine

Chapter 5

Food and your health

Food Technology

Your health is threatened by food technology. Your food is bleached, coloured, dehydrated, homogenized, emulsified, pasteurized and gassed. Over 1,500 non-nutritive substances are added to the food you buy. While each of these additives is tested in isolation for possible harmful effects, such tests make no allowance for the way in which these substances affect each other and thus the human organism when they are ingested together. Some people are more sensitive than others to such artificial agents. The danger to the consumer from food additives can be judged from a notice which was published in the *British Medical Journal*:

> In theory any food additive or colouring shown to cause cancer in animals must be banned. In practice (*Science* 1985:229:739-41) the Food and Drugs Administration is stalling on six commonly used dyes known to be animal carcinogens. Red No. 3, for example, brightens maraschino cherries and many other foods. Since 1981 the FDA (Food and Drugs Administration) has proposed banning it on 12 occasions and each time the dye has been reprieved. Apparently pressure from industry has repeatedly persuaded the commissioners that the risk is 'trivial' - to the outrage of the consumer groups. [1]

Another disturbing example of a possible hazard to health by an additive has recently come to light. It concerns a substance called butylated hydroxyanisole, BHA, shown on food labels as E320. It stops products becoming rancid. Tests, carried out for the Ministry of Agriculture, Fisheries and Food 'suggest that the additive may be a mutagen - capable of causing deformities [[in children]] '. The product has been banned in Japan, but is found in Britian in a great variety of foods: baked goods, sweets, raisins, margarine, and a host of others including beef stocks, packet convenience foods, potato crisps and cooking oils to prevent them from becoming rancid. BHA is combined with another additive, BHT. 'When the two are used together, BHT concentrates the BHA in our body fat to 20 times above normal levels', says Maurice Hanssen, author of the book *New E for Additives*.

The authorities are obviously aware of the danger to children from this substance, as BHA is not allowed in foods which are specifically for babies and young children, but it is certain that this danger is not averted as children consume many of the foods which contain BHA.[2]

The scientific-technological treatment of the white bread that your baker offers you calls for your strongest protest: from the outer layer of the grain its rich mineral and vitamin content has been extracted and the 'heart' of the grain, the wheat germ, has been removed. These are the most nutritious and valuable parts. White bread is then 'enriched' with nine vitamins and a further nine chemicals. The miller adds 'improvers', bleachers, maturing agents - chlorine dioxide being one of them.

While you can avoid eating white bread and can eat wholemeal bread instead, you will have difficulty in avoiding sugar which of course is often added to white flour in the making of cakes, pastries, puddings and other bakeries. It is the main constituent of the enormous variety of sweets and is consumed by technological man in great quantities, the average per person being 5-6 ounces per day! This amount corresponds to 2 lb of sugarbeet (the brown sugar is usually coloured white sugar). Sugar in its natural state is a mixture of glucose, lactose, sucrose and other complex molecules. The food industry has isolated one of these elements, sucrose, a chemically pure substance.

The harmful effects of the consumption of sugar have been explained by a critical nutritional expert:

> Whereas at one time our natural instinctive desire for sugar would lead towards natural sugar-bearing food such as raw fruit, honey, carob, molasses and raw maple syrup which contain plenty of vitamins, minerals and enzymes, our natural hunger is now satisfied with sugary carbohydrate foods which add to body weight and give little or no nutritional benefit.

The same writer blames the food industry for adding flavouring agents to food: 'artificial flavouring has deceived our flavour senses into taking food not good for us'.[3]

Apart from causing obesity, the consumption of sugar and white flour causes tooth decay. An American dentist has shown how the splendid teeth of people living on natural foods decay within one generation once the population is introduced to these refined carbohydrates. Not only are the teeth affected, but the development of the bones in the head is disturbed and possibly also the development of the brain.[4] There are further dangers to your health from eating an excess of refined carbohydrates: they include ulcers in stomach and duodenum, formation of pouches in the large bowel, varicose veins and a state of imbalance of the micro-organisms which inhabit the large bowel. Furthermore, diabetes and atherosclerosis (hardening of arteries) are linked to sugar which accumulates in the blood.

The dangerous degeneration in the artery wall, the atheroma, is of a fatty nature and has also been related to increased consumption of meat from animals which have been reared under modern scientific methods of intensive husbandry. Their meat contains 25-30 per cent fat, whereas a cow, free to select its own food, has been shown to have a carcass fat of 3.9 per cent.[5]

The food industry uses a chemical, nitrate, to preserve meat and also to give a bright red colour to ham and to frankfurters. The serious dangers arising from this substance were stressed in the introductory chapter which was concerned with the relationship of man and his natural environment to the balance in nature.[6] Nitrite, developing from nitrate, has been linked with the formation of cancer which is rising throughout the industrialized world. The cancer-producing properties of nitrates may become active if the person eats substances which combine with nitrites at the same time, but the food industry has neglected research into the effects of food combination, as it adopts the characteristic scientific fragmentary approach which isolates individual chains of causes and effects, leaving out the consideration of the whole. The food industry also neglects to take notice of research which has been carried out in relation to uptake of nitrates into vegetables, which has led to legal enforcements of standards in Switzerland and Holland. In these investigations the nitrate content of samples of celery, lettuce and cress, all on sale to the public, were frequently found to exceed the legal limits in force in Switerzland and Holland. In spring cabbages 'the nitrate content tended to rise coincidental with the time when heavy applications of fertilizers are usually made to the soil on which the crops are grown'.[7]

Apart from neglecting the wholeness of the biological processes in the single individual, food technology also neglects the mutual relations between the living organism and its environment, the ecology. Chemical fertilization has already been criticized, and to this must be added forced cropping which serves financial gain. Overmechanization adds to the imbalance. The soil gets exhausted, crops are devitalized.

Science never stands still. It can now synthesize foods: fat from petroleum, protein from microbes grown in fermentation vessels. We are expected to live on such synthetic food. A critic has complained that

> nutrition science has not investigated the matter further; nothing is known about other qualities of real meat that may be significant to good health and well-being. At least beefsteak is a whole food, whereas soybean meat is a set of extracted molecules divorced from its original context in the soybean. The effects of such a divorce have not been studied, and nutrition scientists seem convinced that the fabricated soybean protein is nutritionally no different from beef protein.[8]

As the same author has pointed out:

> technology founded on mechanistic laws clashes head on with the processes of a natural world which adheres to very different laws. Modern industry, ignoring these biological laws, moulds and manipulates natural processes to suit and to promote its own mechanistic and economic goals .... Mechanization with its reorganization of living processes in the name of human nourishment has resulted in a totally new and contrived biological ideology in which man is processed as much as any other element of the defined system.[9]

Diet and disease

Diseases are treated by scientific medicine specifically which means that causes which explain the disease phenomena are isolated and are then the target for the treatment. Diet is an example. Specific diets are prescribed for instance for obesity, where a reduction of calories is essential, for diabetes where sugar intake has to be related to the patient's ability to deal with it, or for kidney diseases where the protein requirement has to be adjusted to the kidney function.

Natural therapy does not classify patients primarily according to diseases but according to the need for altering their life style which affects the whole person. This does not mean for instance that specific disturbances in kidneys, or in the pancreas which leads to diabetes, and obesity can be ignored. These factors are considered within general unspecific treatment. Although the disease concept is not basic to natural therapy, the following discussion of three diseases from a dietetic point of view will confirm and clarify the principles of natural therapy. The first two diseases, heart disease and cancer, are major killers, the third is not recognized by scientific medicine but represents a true natural therapy point of view and throws light on a number of diseases, treated in isolation from the underlying dietetic fault by scientific medicine. It has been called 'saccharine disease'.

Heart disease
The British Heart Foundation has issued a leaflet about the disease which is characterized by an interference with the blood supply to the heart muscle leading to the death of the affected parts of the heart and frequently to sudden death. The leaflet accepts that inheritance plays some part, but maintains that diet is of vital importance. The emphasis is on reducing the level of the fatty substance, cholesterol, in the blood which is said to be the main factor responsible for the heart disease. Their recommendations are:

1.   Eat less saturated fat which is the fat in meat, meat products and dairy products. It warns against the 'hidden fat' in 'fast foods', such as cakes, biscuits, chocolate. It advises against frying and roasting, as these involve the use of fats. And it promotes the use of vegetable oils such as corn, sunflower and olive in preference to hard fats.

2.   Poultry and fish are to be preferred, meat being suspect because, as we saw, it contains an excessive amount of fat due to the artificial methods of rearing the animals.

3.   More bread, cereal, rice, potatoes and pasta should be consumed, in particular brown bread and brown rice, i.e., wholemeal bread and unpolished rice, the natural unadulterated products. The need to eat more vegetables and fruit which, we shall see, play a major part in the holistic diet advocated by natural therapy, is stressed.

4.   People should eat less sugar which, again, is in accordance with the principles of Natural Therapy, as will be explained later.

5.   Salt, which is often hidden in prepared foods - another example of harmful food technology - should be used less.

Wrong eating habits are not the only cause for heart attacks which were earlier quoted as amounting to 1¼ million per year in America. Smoking of cigarettes and over-consumption of alcohol are major contributors to heart trouble. Smoking and excessive drinking also play their part along with diet in the causation of cancer. The scientific evidence regarding food and cancer will now be reviewed, and will strengthen natural therapy's case.

Cancer

As was stated before, the threat to life and health from cancer can be measured by the figures from America and Great Britain: the figures were an incidence of some 200,000 cases in Britain every year and for America the startling statement that one in every three Americans will get some cancer before reaching 74.

In June 1980 the National Research Council in the United States conducted a comprehensive study of the relationship of diet and nutrition to cancer and added its recommendations related to dietary components including toxic contaminants. [10] The following are some of the findings.

Consumption of foods which were high in so-called saturated fats (derived from animals) in combination with a low intake of fibre was associated with cancer in the large bowel, the breasts and the prostate gland. [11] Natural therapy emphasizes a vegetarian diet (including dairy produce) and a liberal quantity of fibre. Meat-eaters, compared with strict vegetarians, suffer two to three times the risk of developing cancer in the large bowel. Serum cholesterol, comparatively low in vegetarians, was found at higher than usual levels in patients suffering from cancer of the stomach, pancreas, liver, bile ducts and rectum. [12] The rate of breast cancer in women who ate large amounts of animal fats and proteins and small amounts of fibre was higher than in women not eating such a diet. [13]

The role of protein was investigated. 'The incidence of and mortality from breast cancer was significantly correlated with intakes of total protein and animal protein.' [14] Cancers in the large bowel and the rectum were also related to intake of total and animal protein. These findings refute the idea that large amounts of protein, especially meat protein, are health promoting.

Foods containing vitamin A were found to reduce the risk of cancer, but an increase of vitamin A as a supplement was considered to be inadvisable as it can be toxic. This conclusion is in line with the objection, raised earlier, against the prescription of vitamin A supplements. [15]

Vitamin C was found to give some protection against cancers of the stomach and oesophagus, but these findings were related to the consumption of foods containing vitamin C and not to the intake of vitamin C tablets. [16]

No evidence of the effects on cancer by vitamin E and vitamin B were reported. With regard to minerals, supplements of selenium did not show any health benefits. The evidence for dietary zinc was inconclusive. With regard to iron no conclusions were reached. The same applies to copper. There was no evidence regarding iodine and cancer. Exposure to lead may pose a risk of cancer.[17]

The National Research Council also reported on the possible dangers from nitrate and nitrite as a chemical fertilizer and a food preservative.

> Studies conducted in Columbia, Chile, Japan, Iran, China, England, and the United States have indicated that there is an association between increased incidence of cancers of the stomach and the esophagus and exposures to high levels of nitrate or nitrite in the diet or drinking water. Bladder cancer has been correlated with nitrate in the water supply or with urinary tract infections in some epidemiological studies.

Though the evidence was not conclusive, it was, however, 'largely circumstantial'.[18]

The chapter in the report that reviews the protection given by foods against the development of cancer is of particular importance to natural therapy. For it relates that raw vegetables, including coleslaw and red cabbage, are related to a lower risk of stomach cancer. Similar findings are also reported from Japan where lettuce and celery were studied.[19] Natural therapists often prescribe diets of raw vegetables for patients for long periods and, even when cooked foods are added, patients are instructed to eat raw salads every day in sufficiently large quantities. Consumption of vegetables such as cabbage, broccoli, cauliflower and brussels sprouts were found to be associated with a reduction in the incidence of cancer at various sites in human beings.[20] These findings support the practice of natural therapists who recommend the consumption of these vegetables in a cooked form.

Cancer and heart disease are both killers of people who live on processed and unbalanced diets, the result of an artificial man-made ecology. Natural therapy does not use the classification according to disease, but is concerned, rather, with habits or life styles as causing disease. It accepts the term 'disease' as referring to a fault in eating which covers a multitude of 'diseases' in different parts of the body. Such a term is 'saccharine disease'.

Saccharine disease

Two British doctors have coined the term 'saccharine disease'[21] as a single entity which makes the consumption of refined carbohydrates responsible not for a single disease, but for a whole host of diseases. There are grounds for this view. During the last hundred years the western diet has changed radically. One of the changes, the excessive consumption of sugar, has already been criticized. Carbohydrates which provide the foundation of human diet, are processed. The technological treatment of bread was condemned earlier. Most flour is now 'refined' and excessive amounts of sugar are consumed.

This change in eating habits has seriously upset the balance of the whole organism. It is now claimed that not only obesity - the all too obvious result of over-indulgence in sugar and flour - but a whole range of other conditions which plague people today can be recognized as manifestations of the saccharine disease.

There is a connection between the consumption of refined carbohydrates and the loss of sound teeth, but diabetes mellitus should also be looked at in relation to the over-consumption of carbohydrates. The pancreas (the gland which is mainly concerned with sugar metabolism) suffers when having to deal with an excess of carbohydrates, and studies in Natal support this contention. The Indians living there show a frequency of diabetes which is 'one of the highest in the world and probably ten times as high as in India itself - and their sugar consumption is nearly ten times as high too'.[22] Studies have shown that saccharine disease has further manifestations: the refined diet causes unnatural loading of the colon which in turn leads to stasis and pressure on the venous return within the pelvis. Thus, varicose veins in the legs, enlargement of the veins within the scrotum and haemorrhoids are the result. Further proof is again provided by comparing people who live on unrefined foods with those who adopt the habit of food refinement. The two groups show significant differences with regard to the prevalence of ulcers in the stomach and in the duodenum. A connection has been made between these peptic ulcers and the over-consumption of refined carbohydrates: the refined carbohydrates enter the stomach without being accompanied by proteins (which have been eliminated through the refining process). The result is that the acid in the stomach is not neutralized, and this excess of acid contributes to the formation of ulcers.

But the range of saccharine disease extends further and includes coronary disease, in which the significance of tobacco smoking has already been stressed. High carbohydrate consumption has been strongly suggested as a further factor, for coronary disease and obesity are often associated, and diabetes and coronary disease also go hand in hand. Thus, as these two conditions are frequently caused by carbohydrate over-consumption, the inclusion of coronary disease in saccharine illness appears to be justified.

The various manifestations of saccharine disease confirm the natural therapist's conception that the organism functions as a whole, and that an imbalance in the diet has widespread harmful consequences for the whole person. Further confirmation can be found in the fact that over-eating of carbohydrates upsets the equilibrium of the bowel flora - the different types of micro-organisms which are present in the large bowel. This additional disturbance has been considered to be a contributory cause of inflammation of the appendix, the gall bladder and the kidney (pyelitis). All these conditions are common in the west and, by contrast, are extremely rare in those communities which adhere to a diet which does not contain refined carbohydrates.[23]

Lack of dietary fibre

A surplus of refined carbohydrates leads to widespread disease processes; a lack of dietary fibre, often combined with such surplus, leads to other abnormalities in different parts of the body (apart from cancers which have already been dealt with). After a comparison of people who consume a diet rich in fibre content with others whose diets are deficient in fibre, the following conditions have been related to such a deficiency:

Diverticular disease consists in the formation of pouches in the gut which are liable to get inflamed and cause serious symptoms. The condition is extremely common in western countries where fibre is often lacking in the diet. It is rare in societies who consume unrefined foods, rich in fibre. The mechanism of the condition has been explained: a low fibre diet leads to hard stools which when being expelled raise the pressure within the bowel lumen, leading to pouch formation.

Appendicitis is rare in rural parts of Africa and Asia where fibre is plentiful in the diet. The incidence of the disease rose in African troops who started eating refined cereals as part of their army ration. The evidence is that the initial lesion is obstructive, brought about by lack of diet fibre.

Apart from preventing the inflammation of bowel diverticula and appendicitis, dietary fibre has been found to protect people against developing high blood pressure with its serious dangers of a stroke and a heart attack. 'Subjects with a high-fibre intake were found to have lower mean blood pressures than those with a low-fibre intake.'[24]

Serum cholesterol, a causative factor of coronary heart disease, is much lower in adult vegetarians (who consume more fibre than meat eaters) than it is in non-vegetarians. In an article on 'Fibre and disease', the following were added to the list of diseases related to lack of dietary fibre: constipation, irritable bowel syndrome, haemorrhoids, varicose veins, hiatus hernia, diabetes, obesity, coronary heart disease and gallstones. This information was obtained by comparing people who live in countries where the food contains plenty of fibre, with those who consume more fat, sugar and animal protein (especially refined carbohydrates) with a consequent drastic reduction in the consumption of fibre-containing foods such as vegetables, legumes and fruit.[25]

Food allergy

Some people are made ill by food which to most is healthy and is also recommended by natural therapists. Some bodies are sensitive to such items as milk, eggs, wheat, fish, nuts, soya products, citrus fruits and yeast. The list includes tea, coffee and artificial colouring agents which natural therapists do not recommend. The diseases that can be caused by these substances include migraine, diseases of the bowel such as the common irritable bowel syndrome which is characterized by abdominal pain and diarrhoea, Crohn's disease which is an inflammation of the bowel with severe abdominal pain and diarrhoea, other forms of colitis with bloody diarrhoea which may affect young children, painful joints with evidence of rheumatic disorder, bronchial asthma and eczema. Sensitivity to gluten, contained in flour, has been known to exist in a bowel disease, coeliac disease, which also can manifest itself on the skin. Soya bean protein has been found to be responsible for the same symptoms as gluten in some of these patients.

The explanation of these phenomena is that for the sensitive person the particular food acts as an allergen, a substance to which the immune system of the body reacts with symptoms of illness. Efforts to diagnose such allergies by examining the patient's blood or by introducing small amounts of foods into the skin have proved to be unreliable. Thus proof of these allergies can only be obtained by trying out the effects of foods which might cause allergic reactions. This means that items which might provoke a reaction are introduced into the diet. This can be a simple matter if people find out that each time they eat a piece of chocolate or cheese, they suffer an attack of migraine. They know then that they have to avoid such foods. The situation is more difficult if young children must be fed without milk and soya protein because they are sensitive to both. The danger is that they will not receive sufficient nourishment. Some hypersensitive children can be helped if a colouring agent, frequently added to foods in tins and packets and also present in many medicines, has been eliminated. These children benefit physically and emotionally from such treatment.

People may find compliance with the recommended diets very difficult. One report states that out of forty children suffering from eczema, only fourteen continued with their diets. It is reassuring to hear that many milk-sensitive children grow out of their sensitive state by the age of one year, the majority by two years and virtually all by four years. Some infants are even intolerant of breast milk.[26]

Information on diet and disease provides important guidelines. Heart disease and cancer are terrible scourges and rightly greatly feared. Allergic diseases are very troublesome. The information enables patients to avoid a lot of suffering if they follow the guidelines. Natural therapy was found to agree with many of the lessons which our discussion on health and disease has yielded. The time has come to discover how a natural therapist approaches the question of your health in relation to your food. This approach was outlined earlier and must now be applied to dietetics.

As was stressed, natural therapy is not analytical as scientific medicine is. It is holistic which means that it is based on faith in the recuperative power of nature in case of disease. Natural therapy acts by paying attention to the conditions under which the mysterious power of life can operate. Where the conditions appear to be unfavourable, a change is advocated. This change, as was pointed out, acts as a stimulus to this creative holistic power to bring about better health or recovery from illness. In dietetics the change consists in a variety of diets, more or less drastic, so that the organism can be stimulated to respond to attain the desired end. In all this the dietetic treatment differs fundamentally from that prescribed by scientific medicine which is dominated by the mechanistic view of food as the supplier of energy. The example of saccharine disease illustrated the natural therapy approach, making over-eating of carbohydrates the overall cause of different diseases, that is that they are explained by the single cause of unfavourable, unnatural conditions of living. From this negative perspective we now move to a description of diets which act as a stimulus to better functioning.

Individual diets

Milk diet

The Milk Diet achieves elimination of superfluous fluids by stimulating the kidneys. Each day in the course of this regime you drink four glasses of milk, to which one litre of Vichy water or distilled water may be added. On this form of diet, you lose sodium chloride (common salt) through your kidneys.

The Milk Diet can be continued for four days. It has been found beneficial in cases of heart failure with retention of fluid (oedema), but it is also suitable for inflammation of the skin (dermatitis) which is associated with 'weeping', that is the oozing of fluid.

Milk is useful not only to stimulate kidney activity, but also to inhibit bowel action and therefore is used with great benefit in cases of diarrhoea (unless the patient is unable to digest milk). Milk can be made more digestible by adding to it a culture of the lactic acid bacillus, and then incubating it at 55°F (13°C) for six to twelve hours. The same result can be achieved by adding lactic acid, drop by drop, to boiled skimmed milk (up to 45 drops to a pint). Buttermilk, the fluid left over after the milk fat has been removed, also helps cases of diarrhoea and, like milk, is a stimulus to the kidneys.

Grape diet

Whereas milk contains protein, carbohydrates, fats and mineral salts, grapes are rich only in sugar. They also contain certain acids and traces of mineral salts. Eating about four pounds of grapes per day (including the skins, after they have been thoroughly washed to remove the effects of spraying,and also eating some of the pips) for several weeks has been of remarkable benefit. People who had been suffering from a variety of complaints, including those of the liver and joints, have reported great improvement and generally feel that their bodies have been cleansed. Their kidneys and bowels are stimulated to eliminate waste and toxins. The grape cure is one of the dietetic treatments which help the whole body and which tend to restore your health.

Fasting on water and fruit juices

In natural therapy, the fast is the most dramatic way of making a change in dietetic habits. Apart from the emotional response, the physical effects vary from person to person. The results of fasting have been measured from time to time, and one such study, carried out by two medical scientists, examined the weight losses and changes in the various constituents of the body.[27] The subjects were 58 female and 18 male patients and the duration of the fast extended over more than 14 days. There was a rapid loss of weight in the first two weeks. Amongst the women, the highest figure was that of a woman of 51 who reduced her original weight of 117.4 kg by 11 kg (1 st 10 lb). The lowest figure was shown in the case of a woman of 34 whose weight went down from 122.1 kg by only 1.34 kg (3 lb). On average, men lost more weight than women during the first two weeks; after that, the mean losses for the two sexes were similar. The differences were attributed to different amounts of water excretion by the kidneys, but were also explained on the basis of different losses of physical activity. Patients showed different losses of the mineral potassium. This should be supplied during a fast. It can be given in fruit juices or as potassium salt.

Another scientific study, carried out on very fat people, found that no harmful effects were noted during the phase of initial rapid weight loss, and that there was prompt improvement in people who had serious respiratory or cardiac conditions. Common early side-effects were mild headache, occasional nausea and some nervous tension. People became less fit physically, but young ones maintained their vigour better than older patients. Sleep patterns were not affected, but sensitivity to cold was increased. The blood pressure dropped after the third and fourth weeks, and with this drop came a rise in pulse rate and a feeling of weakness leading to a sensation of faintness in some patients. The level of uric acid rose, causing attacks of gout in two patients.

Starvation was considered to be a strain on the heart, and a drop in blood pressure was thought to be dangerous to people who had recently suffered from a heart attack (myocardial infarction). Other people who were not thought suitable for fasting included those with a history of anaemia, liver disease or inadequate circulation of the heart (coronary insufficiency manifest in attacks of angina pectoris). The sufferers from gout required the addition of protein.

When blood pressure dropped, patients were given food. Vitamins were required throughout. Three men developed anaemia in the second month (the experiment lasted sixty days).[28]

These experiments not only provide a natural therapist with some valuable information, but also highlight the difference between natural therapy and the conventional medical approach. The natural therapist distinguishes between fasting and starvation. There is no therapeutic *starvation,* according to natural therapy; there is only therapeutic *fasting*. This difference has been explained in the following terms: 'To *fast* is to abstain from food while one possesses adequate reserves to nourish vital tissues; to *starve* is to abstain from food after reserves have been exhausted so that vital tissues are sacrificed.'[29]

While the conventional physician sees a reason for withholding food only in cases of obesity, the natural therapist sees, in fasting, a most potent way of giving the body a chance of recovering from the disequilibrium which disease in general represents. The loss of weight is only incidental, although it figures prominently in cases of overweight. To the natural therapist, fasting means giving the organism a rest so that repair work can be carried out. Digestion puts a strain on the stomach and the intestines, on the liver, the pancreas and on all the glands which deal with the assimilation of food. The work load is slowed down during abstinence from food, which means a rest also for other functions of the body, such as respiration and nervous activity. At the same time, the mind is at rest - provided the surroundings are peaceful.

The experience of a fast can be of vital importance in your life. It can be a turning point in your attitude towards values; you can recognize and correct your tendency to over-eat, to rely on alcohol, smoking, tea and coffee. This can be the time when you come to accept responsibility for your health. Fasting is a time for stocktaking.

A patient who is frightened of the effects of fasting, or who is surrounded by well-meaning people who warn him against abstinence from food, saying that it will be dangerous to his health, cannot benefit from a fast. Therefore, fasts are often taken in a home where other patients are having the same experience, and where the staff are experienced in handling the treatment. Under the guidance of an experienced natural therapist, you should feel safe and assured that the fast will be correctly terminated.

The fast is a cleansing process which may be experienced in the following way: your therapist interprets the bad breath and the coated tongue which are always present at the beginning of the fast as evidence of toxic eliminations. You are not hungry after the first two days; but you may feel sick and may actually vomit or have diarrhoea - further efforts on the part of your body to get rid of unwanted matter. You may complain of a headache - a manifestation of your toxic condition.

Gradually your appetite returns, the tongue clears and your breath becomes sweet: then the fast can be broken. During the fast, you should be allowed to rest as much as you desire. You should be comfortably warm; lukewarm sponges of your body and mild sun baths are helpful.

In an article on regeneration during a fast and while taking juices, Dr E. Heun has summarized the results of many investigations. He holds that destruction of unhealthy tissue through fasting must precede the building-up of sound cells through the taking of whole-food. Heun has classified the various tissues with regard to their capacity to regenerate: the cells of the blood and lymph, the bone marrow and lymphatic organs re-form quickly, so do the liver cells and those cells which line the inner organs, as well as the elements which form the skin. Muscle and nerve cells show much less capacity for regrowth; the cells in the brain do not grow again after they have been destroyed. During a fast, shrinking occurs in the above order of regeneration, leaving the most valuable tissues intact. Substances which are released during the death of cells stimulate the growth of new cells. This constructive process is initiated during a fast, leading to rejuvenation of the whole organism, but with advancing age the power of regeneration diminishes.

Heun has traced the changes of the cells in the blood through the various stages and has followed their defensive actions against the toxins in the body throughout the fast. He attributes to the lymph a scavenging role. The skin looks younger after the fast, as its circulation has improved. The inner linings of the body take part in the cleansing process which is visible on the tongue, but is also evident in the intestinal and urinary tracts from the appearance of mucous secretions found in the stools and in the urine. There is regeneration of the thyroid gland, the ovaries and the testes, as well as in other parts of the body which are concerned with regulation of vital processes. At the end of his article, Heun discusses 'psychocatharsis', a spiritual regeneration, a 'digestion' of pent-up emotional waste. [30]

Fasting is beneficial in acute and in chronic disease. Any acute condition - a cold, an attack of bronchitis, of tonsilitis, any of the children's diseases such as measles - is best treated by a fast; that is, by giving only water or fruit juice to the patient. In this way the body recovers without having to cope with the toxic side-effects of such drugs as aspirin, or having to waste energy on the digestion of food. In fact, the natural instinct, when acutely ill, is to abstain from food. A sick animal does not eat when ill. In cases of chronic disease the natural therapist has to assess the patient's ability to respond bodily and mentally to fasting.

Many sufferers from such chronic diseases as rheumatoid arthritis, bronchial asthma and inflammation of the kidneys, benefit from a well-conducted fast. Patients who are unsuitable, from whom no response can be expected, are the very young, the very old and those who suffer from some debilitating disease such as cancer, or a chronic disease of the nervous system. In cases of gastric and duodenal ulcer, fasting may precipitate a haemorrhage and is therefore too dangerous.

The fast is broken by introducing the next grade of the natural dietetic stimulus: the raw fruit and raw vegetable regime.

Raw fruit and vegetable diet

After a fast, a diet consisting of raw fruits and raw vegetables is the next step in the stimulation of the body by dietetic means. Raw fruit and vegetables contain enzymes (elements which bring about necessary chemical changes in the body) which are destroyed by cooking and processing. As Shears has pointed out: 'In order to help furnish the body with the elements which it needs, they must necessarily be obtained in organic life-containing form as in raw vegetables and in particular in the form of fresh vegetables and fruit juices.'[31]

Fresh fruit and vegetables also contain, in concentrated form, vitamins needed by the body. These are related to one another; therefore the taking of single vitamins can easily upset the balance. Fresh fruits and raw vegetables are alkaline-producing foods, since they form alkaline residues (ashes) and, as such, they counter the acid-forming foods such as meat, eggs, fish, cheese and game. Sugar and flour are also acid-forming. These acid-forming substances are taken to excess by many people, and the raw fruit and vegetable diet acts an an antidote. Natural therapists believe that, in order to keep well, we need a surplus of alkaline-producing foods and that people who follow a conventional diet suffer from an upset of their acid/alkaline balance.

A raw fruit and raw vegetable diet may consist of the following items: for breakfast, muesli (oats soaked overnight, mixed with a grated apple and a little lemon juice and nut cream); for lunch and for supper, raw vegetables, nuts, olive oil. Dried or fresh fruits are added to the salads.

The patients of conventional physicians are only rarely given the benefit of this type of diet, as medical training does not provide the student with the necessary conception of a sick body responding favourably to the stimulus of a raw fruit and raw vegetable diet. To the ordinary doctor, the overriding dietetic concern is the calorific need, and the supply of the various elements (protein, carbohydrates, fats, vitamins and mineral salts) in sufficient quantities.

Dr D.C. Hare of the Royal Free Hospital in London took an exceptional step in 1936 by feeding patients suffering from osteoarthritis, acute rheumatoid arthritis, chronic rheumatoid arthritis, and 'muscular rheumatism', on one pint of milk, raw fruit, raw vegetables and Bircher-Benner Muesli made with 90 gm (3 oz) of cream. There was a remarkable improvement, a relief of pain and, in eight out of twelve patients, the joints became less stiff and less swollen. Alas, after only two weeks Dr Hare added eggs, cheese and meat.[32] Later, the trial was repeated by Drs Hare and Pillman-Williams on six patients suffering from rheumatoid arthritis; five of them benefited although the sixth disappeared.[33]

Unlike a physician such as Dr Hare, a natural therapist, when applying the dietetic stimulus, is not guided by a diagnosis or by the concern to meet a patient's calorific or nutritional needs. He observes the response and, in many cases, keeps the patient on a reduced diet for weeks and months, with excellent results. He is encouraged by the reports published in scientific medical literature which confirm the fallacy of considering the human person in terms of a combustion engine.

A striking example has been given in Sweden. Twelve men, aged 20 to 50, walked 50 km (about 31 miles) per day for ten days while their diet was restricted to mineral water, apple juice, orange and grape juice, and freshly prepared carrot and red beet juice. They also took vitamin and mineral tablets. Each man's total daily calorific intake was 340, whereas his calculated needs would have been well over 3,000. In spite of this 'deficiency', they remained perfectly well.[34] During a longer period, extending over several months, a Japanese doctor proved that he and his wife could maintain excellent health on raw whole rice, raw vegetables and a little fruit.[35]

Full diet

(A) ESSENTIAL COMPONENTS

After you have been living on a restricted diet and have eliminated toxins, the natural therapist will proceed to build up a diet to satisfy your body's permanent needs. Depending on your case, the full diet may be prescribed sooner or later in the treatment. Many people who are not fit for a strict diet because they are too old or too young, or those who are not suffering from a serious condition which would justify a drastic change, start with a full diet. But what is a full diet to one person, who maintains his weight on it, is an eliminative diet to another. The result depends on whether the digestive organs are able to extract the necessary nourishment from the food. It is common experience in natural therapy that the same amount and combination of ingredients can lead to an initial loss of weight in a person who, later on, maintains his weight or even increases it. In the course of time his organs have acquired the ability to assimilate the food.

The natural therapist must consider an individual's likes and dislikes. To force down food which does not appeal is useless; it will not be digested properly, as the digestive juices only flow when food is wanted.

A balance of ingredients is vital. This balance is best safe-guarded by eating food grown in healthy soil and eaten whole and fresh whenever possible. We shall now briefly discuss the items which make up a full diet.

Protein. The protein should be derived from wholegrain cereals, pulses and dairy produce. Meat and fish are for those who cannot accept a lacto-vegetarian diet, even though it supplies all the necessary protein. The soya bean is a very good source of protein, as are nuts, seeds, avocados, almonds and yeast. People engaged in strenuous exercise require extra protein. The minimum need has been estimated to be 0.5 gm protein per kilo bodyweight.

Carbohydrate. Wholegrain, compost-grown bread, cereals such as wheat, oats, barley, rice and maize; potatoes; honey and sweet fruits such as dates, figs and grapes: these are the main sources of carbohydrate. Beetroot and root vegetables, for instance, turnips and carrots, yield further supplies and so does milk, which contains milk sugar. Pulses (peas, beans and so on) provide starches as well as proteins.

Fat. Cream and butter, margarine (which may be made from animal or vegetable fat), olive oil, almond oil and nuts, are the main sources of fat.

The Royal College of Physicians and the British Cardiac Society have recently warned against the customary fat consumption which amounts to 42 per cent of all calories. The report insists that this high figure is an important factor in the incidence of heart disease which is particularly prevalent in Britain. The proportion of fat should be reduced to at least 35 per cent and 'polyunsaturated' fats, such as corn and sunflower seed oil or safflower oil should replace as far as possible the fat which is obtained from meat, butter, cream, milk and fatty cheeses. Olive oil is also preferable to cream. It can be diluted with polyunsaturated oil as a salad dressing. The natural therapist accepts these recommendations.

Vitamins. The following tables summarize the role played by vitamins in the body and indicate the sources of supply:

Vitamin	Sources of supply
A: Deficiency leads to diseases of the eye, the skin and the linings of internal organs. The vitamin is stored in the liver and feverish diseases can depress the store. Nitrate, used as a preservative for sausages, salami and other foods such as frankfurters, hamburgers and canned meat, also depresses the vitamin A stores in the liver.	Milk, butter, eggs, liver, fish and fish oils. In a preliminary state it occurs in carrots, turnip tops, spinach, parsley, watercress, cabbage and lettuce.
B1: A deficiency of this vitamin is known to cause a great many symptoms such as fatigue, depression, dizziness, sore muscles, palpitation, chest pain, sleeplessness, loss of appetite and weight, vomiting, weakness of muscles, irregular heartbeats and low blood pressure. The body's vitamin B1 requirements are raised by the ingestion of excessive amounts of sugar. The refining of flour destroys a large percentage of this vitamin which is essential for growth and for the proper functioning of the heart, nerves and muscles.	Wholemeal bread, unpolished rice, oatmeal, milk, yeast, butter beans, haricot beans, peas, lentils, meat and eggs.
B2: This vitamin is needed to promote healthy conditions of skin, mouth and hair and is essential for the functioning of the eyes. Without this vitamin, important biochemical transformations in the body cannot take place.	Meat, fish, green vegetables, potatoes, wholegrain products and brewers' yeast.
B3 (Niacin): Essential for the processes which take place in the	Wholegrain flour, unpolished rice, meat and yeast. To a lesser degree it

Vitamin	Sources of supply
intestinal tract, in the skin and the nervous system. Vitamin B3 is not present in white flour or in polished rice.	is also present in fruit, vegetables, milk and other dairy products.
B6 (Pyridoxine): This vitamin is concerned in many processes connected with the building of body tissues. Its absence leads to such serious consequences as anaemia and neuritis. Individuals vary in their requirement of it.	Widely distributed in food.
B12 (Cyanocobalamin): A deficiency of this vitamin leads to a form of anaemia (pernicious anaemia) which is characterized by complications in the nervous system and by abnormal mental functioning. Vegans, who, as a matter of principle, abstain from all dairy produce (as well as meat and fish), are liable to suffer from vitamin B12 deficiency and have to consider taking this vitamin as a drug.	Foods of animal origin.
Folic Acid: A deficiency is responsible for anaemia.	Green vegetables, liver, meat and fish.
C: Essential for cell activity. Deficiency of this vitamin leads to scurvy, characterized by haemorrhages into the skin and internal organs. Bleeding gums are also a sign of this condition. Deficiency results largely from the degradation of food, and it has been estimated that there is a deficient intake of vitamin C in 54 per cent of British households during the	Fruit and vegetables, especially oranges and other citrus fruits. Also in the green leaves of vegetables and in *unheated* milk.

Vitamin	Sources of supply
winter months and in 25 per cent of British households over the whole year.[36]	
D: This vitamin is formed in the skin by the action of sunlight, which confirms the value of sunbathing. Vitamin D is essential for the formation of a healthy bone structure in children and for maintaining it in adults. The lack of it appears in the bent bones of the rickety child and of the adult who suffers from osteomalacia or bone softening. Extra Vitamin D is required in diseases of the gut and kidneys.	Milk, liver and egg yolk.
E: A controversial vitamin, claimed by some to be important for the proper functioning of the heart and blood vessels, but others deny that it plays any useful part in the human body at all.	Sunflower seed oil, wheatgerm oil, almonds, walnuts and soya-bean oil.
K: This vitamin is made by micro-organisms in the bowel and is lacking in the body if these normal bowel bacteria are destroyed by antibiotics. This confirms the importance of healthy bowel flora for general health, and points to one of the dangers arising from antibiotics. It is essential for the clotting of blood and for the functioning of the liver.	Widely distributed in the plant kingdom. The lacto-vegetarian diet recommended by natural therapists supplies it in ample amounts.

Apart from gross vitamin deficiencies, causing severe symptoms, we have to consider marginal vitamin deficiencies. These may well be responsible for decreased vitality and diminished resistance to disease. There is evidence that some people lack vitamins B1, B6 and C, and that the young and the old need extra amounts of these vital substances. As has been pointed out, the full natural diet preserves vitamins by insisting that food should be raw if possible, and certainly never over-cooked.

Mineral salts. Apart from water, protein, carbohydrates, fat and vitamins, a full diet must contain correct amounts of mineral salts. These will now be discussed.

Iron. Women lose iron with menstrual bleeding and they must therefore have extra supplies. Vitamin C facilitates the absorption of iron from the gut; thus, a lack of this vitamin can cause iron deficiency. Iron is present in meat, cereals, eggs and vegetables.

Wholemeal bread is much richer in iron than white bread, and bran is a rich source. The diet recommended by the natural therapist supplies enough of this mineral.

Magnesium. Your body can adjust itself to a low magnesium intake by absorbing magnesium from the bowels and by restricting its excretion in the urine. Magnesium can prevent the formation of stones in the kidneys and is of importance for general health. Many people have been found to lack sufficient amounts of it. It is removed in the refining of wholegrain cereals and in cooking of vegetables. (Thus, again, the principles of natural therapy are vindicated.) Magnesium is found in wholegrain cereals, nuts, raw vegetables, legumes, and also in seafood and in meat.

Calcium. As with magnesium, the body can adapt itself to a low calcium intake, but there is grave danger in a low calcium diet, for calcium is needed for the formation and maintenance of bones and for the normal excitability of tissues. In severe calcium deficiency there is twitching of muscles. Calcium is needed (with iron) for the manufacture of blood pigment. Cereals, fruit, vegetables and milk provide calcium.

Sodium. Sodium is taken in the form of sodium chloride - table salt. As sodium chloride holds water, a deficiency will lead to a reduction in the volume of body fluids, including blood. The symptoms are fainting, weakness, dizziness, mental confusion, fall in blood pressure, and muscular cramps. As sodium chloride is lost in sweat, a sufficient supply is especially necessary in hot climates and during physical exertion. The natural therapist provides salt for patients undergoing heat treatment which encourages profuse perspiration - but, as we shall see later, even a cold compress can lead to perspiration, and may result in a deficit of sodium chloride in the body.

There is salt in most butter and bread, in sauces, and in preserved and canned meat. People also add salt to their food in cooking and at the table, usually more than is required by their bodies. A low salt diet is valuable in several types of diseases of the kidneys, the heart, and the liver, but people generally find severe salt restriction difficult to bear. The kidneys can protect the body from loss of salt by excreting salt-free urine, and the ordinary evaporation of water from the skin does not contain salt either. Too much salt can be harmful, especially to babies and infants (for whom there is a danger of developing high blood pressure).

Potassium. Potassium is found in most natural whole-foods, for animal and plant cells are rich in it. Fruit juices are a good source of potassium. Potassium deficiency arises from losses associated with vomiting and diarrhoea. In some kidney diseases, and in wasting diseases where cells break down, potassium losses occur. The symptoms are muscle weakness, dizziness, thirst, mental confusion, and interference with the normal excitability of tissues.

Interference with mineral metabolism. The industrial development of our times has introduced harmful elements such as lead, tin, cadmium, fluoride, mercury and arsenic into the human body. These can interfere with the normal mineral metabolism, and may cause disease and deficiencies. Modern agricultural practices have led to the use of mineral fertilizers, such as lime. This may further upset the natural balance, especially of the trace elements, which play an important part in the body.

Trace elements.
Iodine. Iodine is an essential component of the body, and is found in the thyroid gland. Its absence in food leads to the formation of goitre. Iodine is present in seafoods, including fish. People vary in their need for iodine. To give an excess is dangerous for people who suffer from an over-activity of the thyroid gland. Iodine and other substances are found in kelp which is made from seaweed.

Copper. Copper is present in most foods, and high intakes are absorbed from seafood, meat, eggs, nuts, fruit and cereals. Copper facilitates vital processes. On the whole, deficiency is not likely.

Molybdenum. Molybdenum is another essential trace element. It helps to prevent dental caries, and deficiency of this element in the soil makes plants susceptible to fungus infections. There seems to be a danger that the breakdown products from such plant disease can cause cancer in people who eat the diseased plants.[37]

Zinc. Zinc occurs in seafoods, meat, wholegrain products, dairy produce, nuts and legumes but not much in other vegetables. Zinc deficiency has been diagnosed in the Middle East, but not in the West. (As the result of zinc deficiency, children in Iran have failed to mature normally.) This metal is important for the production of sperm, for the growth of bones, and for certain biochemical processes. Zinc aids the healing of wounds. It is related to copper and calcium. Often, as a result of mechanization and the neglect of organic manuring, the soil has become deficient in zinc in many countries, and this fact may have a harmful effect upon human health.

In general, trace elements are refined out of cereals and, as already indicated, agricultural methods can deprive the soil of these important and not fully investigated substances.

(B) A SIMPLE BALANCED DIET

After having defined and evaluated the components which are necessary for a balanced natural diet, we have now to indicate how meals should be planned. Of course, people are expected to choose foods they like, and leave out foods they dislike.

When planning daily menus, note that raw fruit and vegetables (discussed in an earlier section) play a very important part in a full and regular diet. At least 50 per cent of food should consist of raw salads and raw ripe fruit.

Breakfast. Breakfast should be light since, early in the day, your stomach is not ready for much food. The food consumed on the previous day provides the energy needed for the morning; a heavy breakfast only uses up energy in digestion. Breakfast may consist of ripe fruit and yoghurt, or the muesli mixture recommended as part of the raw vegetable diet. The muesli can be made more nourishing by the addition of nuts, sweet almonds, honey, froment or wheat germ, and the fruit content can be varied. The protein in the mixture may be cream or milk, but yoghurt is better. Nut cream and almond cream are also suitable forms of protein and either can replace the dairy produce. Bran (coarse or All Bran) can be added if you are inclined to be constipated. Dried fruit, soaked overnight, and eaten with bran and yoghurt is another breakfast variation.

Lunch. Lunch should consist of a large salad meal in which leaves, roots and fruits are mixed. A dressing of olive oil and lemon juice is better than the conventional salad cream. Wholemeal bread, or some form of crispbread such as Ryvita, with vegetarian margarine and cheese, can be added or, in place of the crispbread, a potato baked in its skin. Nuts can be included as a further source of protein. The salad should be eaten as soon as the vegetables have been cut or grated, as the Vitamin C content is quickly lost when the finely shredded components are exposed to the air. Different types of graters can be used to vary texture and the mixture can include any fresh fruit that is in season and any vegetables, such as lettuce, watercress, celery, onions, leeks, tomatoes, endive, sea-kale, carrots, brussels sprouts, cabbage and red cabbage (both to be finely shredded), beetroot (not prepared in vinegar), radishes, spinach, cucumber, and avocado. Herbs can be added - either fresh (if available) or dried. (When including cheese, note that cottage cheese is more easily digested than other cheeses and that salted cheeses are less advisable than unsalted ones. Strong cheeses are not as good for most people as mild ones.)

Supper (dinner). The third meal includes fresh fruit but also cooked food. Cooked vegetables should be taken. To supply protein, eggs and cheese can be added to the vegetables, or nut and soya dishes can be prepared. (For those who do not wish to be lacto-vegetarians, meat or fish is included.) Potatoes should be baked in their skins or steamed. Salt should be used sparingly. As dessert, fruit is greatly preferable to puddings.

Drinking. Liquids should not be taken with meals as they dilute the gastric juices, but they can be taken before or about two hours after eating. For reasons which have been pointed out, ordinary tea and coffee are not recommended; they should be replaced by herb teas, dandelion coffee, and fruit juices.

Additions
Here is a brief survey of some of the items that can be added to the standard diet to provide choice and variety and here are also warnings of the dangers to health from some of the foods.

Milk A milk diet was described earlier as a short-time measure to stimulate the kidneys and to inhibit over-activity of the bowel. We shall now consider habitual taking of milk from the natural therapist's viewpoint. Milk is an essential food for babies whose mothers cannot breastfeed. It is, however, harmful to some babies, especially to those who are allergic to it; in such cases, it can provoke eczema and must be replaced by substitutes. These are mainly derived from vegetables; for instance, preparations made from soya and nuts.

In the adult population, milk is consumed by many who seem to tolerate it well. It is a food which contains protein, sugar, carbohydrates and mineral salts, especially calcium and phosphorus. As milk relieves indigestion, and as some people develop a strong taste for it, excessive quantities, several pints a day, are being consumed. But there are serious dangers for such people. The natural therapist is concerned with balance, and drinking several glasses of milk upsets the dietetic equilibrium. Evidence of harm from drinking large amounts of milk comes mainly from investigation into the milk consumption of people who develop heart disease, the great modern killer. Some of the patients investigated had earlier suffered from ulcers in the stomach or the duodenum. In those who had been treated with a milk diet, it was found that the frequency of myocardial infarcts was double the frequency found in those who were not so treated or who had not suffered from ulcers. In a series of fourteen consecutive cases of acute myocardial infarct, nine admitted that they had been in the habit of drinking one pint of milk a day, or more.[38] A number of medical scientists investigating the blood of those who had consumed large quantities of milk found that the body had acted against the cream in the milk by producing 'antibodies'. When these were present, the mortality from a myocardial infarction increased 'almost threefold'.[39]

Not only the heart, but also other organs can suffer from excessive milk consumption. B. Jacobson has drawn attention to the serious hazards entailed in adding daily one pint of milk to a mixed diet. This overloads the body with calcium, phosphorus and protein. The body has to break down the protein, and this leads to the formation of oxalate, a substance which is precipitated in the urine as a stone. Jacobson observed that, between 1965 and 1974, the oxalate content of stones found in men and women increased by over 50 per cent and the number of patients treated in the Leeds area in Britain increased fivefold. For this serious state of affairs, he blames the drinking of milk (shown, on average, to amount to 4.79 pints (2.7 litres) per week per person in Great Britain during 1973-4.[40]

Over-consumption of milk causes not only disturbances in the heart and in the urinary tract; the resulting imbalance leads also to disturbances in other organs. In one community which made milk almost its staple food many suffered from angina pectoris, from a tendency to congestion of the lungs, from inflammation and enlargement of the tonsils and inflammation of the middle ear. When milk was eliminated from the diet and replaced by fruits, vegetables (especially soya), nuts and seafoods, all these disturbances disappeared;[41] the fact that they were largely catarrhal supports the experience of natural therapists, that milk can be responsible for the formation of mucus in sensitive people.

Eggs Eggs are another good source of protein (twelve grammes in a boiled or poached egg). They are also rich in vitamins. But, just like milk, eggs (in their yolk) contain a high amount of cholesterol, a substance which is involved in hardening of the arteries (atherosclerosis). The natural therapist recommends only about three eggs a week. They are to be avoided by people threatened with or suffering from heart trouble and by those who are allergic to them.

Honey Honey consists of a variety of sugars, and because of its concentrated carbohydrate content should be eaten sparingly. It also contains valuable mineral salts, in which darker honey is richer than the light variety.

Soya beans Soya beans are rich in protein and fat, iron and vitamins. They should be cooked and a number of soya products are on the market. Brewers' yeast is rich in those amino-acids (the constituents of protein), which are low in the soya bean. Hence the addition of a little brewers' yeast to a soya dish makes up the deficiency.

Rice Rice is a valuable food which should be taken in the unpolished form. Nutritional losses are incurred by the conventional milling of rice, to the extent that one-third of the protein is lost by the process. By contrast, handpounding cuts out much of this loss (which in the case of refined flour, is the loss of most of the bran).[42] As mentioned earlier, unpolished rice contains the important vitamin B1; the polished product, which has been deprived of the inner husk, is devoid of this vitamin. (Its absence in the diet leads to the disease known as beri-beri which can be cured by substituting unpolished brown rice for white polished rice.)

Sprouting grains In the process of sprouting, grains not only gain enormously in vitamin content but also supply first-class proteins. One study quotes the following impressive analysis of sprouting wheat seeds:

> Sprouting wheat seeds have been analyzed and found to contain 30 per cent more vitamin B; 200 per cent more vitamin B2; 90 per cent more niacin (vitamin B3); 30 per cent more pentothenic acid; and 100 per cent more biotin and pyridoxine (all components of the vitamin B complex) than dormant wheat seeds. During germination, vitamin C is increased by 60 per cent in cereals and germinating soya beans are so rich in vitamin C that a tablespoon of them supplies up to half an adult's daily requirements.

The same author also quotes Dr Francis Pottenger Jr, who 'found that sprouted grains and legumes provided enough first quality proteins to be classed as "complete"'.[43]

It is essential to buy seeds which have not been treated with fungicides such as mercury. The technical details of how to use wheat and rye grains (the commonest varieties) are as follows: the cleansed wheat or rye grains are used either separately or mixed in equal quantities. They are completely covered with water in a container and left overnight with a lid on. The next morning the water is poured off and the grain is left. In the evening fresh water is used to cover the grains. This procedure is continued until the sprouts are visible and have reached the length of a quarter of an inch (6 mm) (they must not be allowed to get bigger). During the process of sprouting, the grains become softer, so that they can be chewed comfortably.

The sprouting should take about three days. In the morning and evening the grains are put into a strainer and rinsed thoroughly with fresh water to remove the yeast and acidity which have developed. The spouting grains can be eaten mixed with milk, rolled oats, and honey or sweet fruits. One to two tablespoonsful of linseed or nuts can also be added. An average daily quantity is two to ten ounces (56-280 grammes) of sprouted grains.

Seeds (unsprouted) Several edible seeds make valuable additions to the diet without having to germinate. Sesame seeds are an example. Once grown by the Romans, they are now cultivated in America, and 'the outstanding characteristic' is the high content of calcium, and of protein -

> between 19 and 28 per cent more than many meats .... Sesame also contains an ample amount of lecithin ⟦ a fatty substance which is an essential element of the cells composing the body ⟧ .... It is especially

rich in two B vitamins ... as well as niacin. Finally sesame is a good source of vitamin E. Sesame seeds form an alkaline rather than an acid reaction within the body.

The seeds can be incorporated in baked foods or combined with honey, or they can be mixed into vegetable dishes. Liquefied sesame seed can be made into sesame milk and can be added to many foods.

Pumpkin seeds are held by one German doctor to be a specific remedy for prostatic enlargement, which is very prevalent among men over the age of 50. This theory is confirmed by the examination of people in places (for instance Transylvania) where the seeds are eaten. These people are said to excel in virility and also to be free from prostatic troubles. An analysis of pumpkin seeds reveals a high content of phosphorus, iron, zinc, B vitamins, protein and fat (in the form of unsaturated fatty acids).[44]

Sunflower seeds are a very rich source of protein, vitamins, minerals, fats and vitamin E, and they also contain iron. They are high in fibre and thus promote the formation of bulky stools, acting against any tendency to constipation.

Avocado pears Avocado pears contain 8 per cent fat, considerable amounts of sodium, potassium, calcium and phosphorus, and some iron and copper, and they are also rich in vitamins. Not only are they a most nourishing food, but they are also protected against contamination by sprays by their thick skins.

Meat and fish or vegetarian or vegan diets?
Most people consider that a meal should contain meat and/or fish. The ordinary family considers these items to be essential and the usual restaurant serves these foods as a matter of course. Many natural therapists either restrict meat and fish dishes to a minimum or advocate a diet which contains dairy produce and eggs as well as the items which have been listed as additions. Some natural therapists go further and recommend a vegan diet which omits dairy produce, eggs and honey as well - in short all foods derived from the animal kingdom. The question arises of whether a vegetarian or vegan diet can be justified and the following aspects must be considered:

HEALTH
The American Dietetic Association has examined the vegetarian approach to eating from a health point of view and other organizations

have come to conclusions similar to theirs. It is important that a vegetarian diet be well planned. Lacto-ovo and lacto-vegetarian diets can meet all the energy requirements. If there has been too great a dependence on milk, iron deficiency is likely. There is a theoretical problem of zinc deficiency. A vegan diet poses the following problems. Children may require fortified soya milk which takes the place of cow's milk. Vitamin D deficiency can occur in children reared on vegan diets if they are not sufficiently exposed to sunlight which enables them to make vitamin D. They may require vitamin D additions, for example synthetic preparations such as Adexolin which contains Vitamins A and D.

Vitamin B12 is lacking in a vegan diet. It can be added in the form of supplements such as Barmene or Granolac or Plamil. Many vegans have been found to manage without Vitamin B12 addition. The health of vegetarians and vegans is often superior to that of meat-eaters. Vegetarians and vegans have a lower incidence of coronary heart disease, which is related to the consumption of fat derived from animals. A study of Seventh-Day Adventists has been illuminating: the risk of fatal coronary heart disease amongst non-vegetarian men aged 35 to 64 years was three times greater than in a group of vegetarian men of comparable age. The incidence of cancer, especially in the stomach and in the large bowel, was lower in the vegetarians than in the meat-eaters. On the whole, vegetarians were found to be less obese than the meat eaters. Important information was gathered with regard to a disease which affects millions of women: osteoporosis, characterized by bones becoming brittle and liable to break on account of loss of calcium. This condition arises when women reach the menopause, when their hormones which cause regular menstruation normally cease to function. At present the policy is to provide those at risk with artificial hormone replacement which, however, is not without risks and in any case only defers the manifestation of the disease by ten years. The investigation, published by the American Dietetic Association, suggests that long-term high-protein intakes lead to negative calcium balance and probably to bone loss. Several authors found that 'lacto-ovo-vegetarians have about half the bone loss after age sixty years experienced by omnivores. The significant difference in bone mineral mass between lacto-ovo-vegetarians and omnivores seen in sixty - to eighty-nine-year-old subjects may in part be diet related.' These findings confirm the disadvantages to health which arise from excessive protein intake which some people consider to be beneficial. Protein is normally derived from meat and fish.[45]

A vegetarian diet, when adopted by meat-eaters, has been found to reduce blood pressure[46] and vegetarians have on the whole lower blood pressures than meat-eaters. High blood pressure is related to heart disease and strokes.

Vegetarians consume more dietary fibre than meat-eaters. A study found that vegetarians get through 41.5 grammes of fibre every day whereas meat-eaters only 21.4 grammes.[47] High-fibre diets are beneficial in many diseases, and protect against cancer of the intestine, diverticular disease[48] and Crohn's Disease.[49] They help towards a remission in ulcerative colitis[50] and in the control of diabetes.[51] The diets of meat-eaters, on account of their high fat and low fibre contents, are thought to contribute towards cancer of the pancreas, breast, ovary, prostate and womb.[52]

A study, carried out at Guy's Hospital in London, revealed that the lower content of protein in vegetarian and vegan diets, compared with that of meat-eaters, has a protective influence on part of the kidneys, the glomeruli, engaged in the production of urine. The increased protein of meat leads to a hardening of these structures which is an important factor in ageing and in a number of kidney diseases. 'These results valuably confirm the benefits of vegetarianism in the maintenance of kidney function and in the repair of defects.'[53]

ECONOMY

A vegetarian or vegan diet is not only healthier than one which also contains meat and fish, it is also far more economical for the individual and for the whole world. Meat and fish are more expensive than milk products, seeds and grains. In addition, meat is a very wasteful way of feeding people. Many poor countries live largely on vegetarian diets, as they cannot afford the luxury of meat production. Ninety per cent of the cereals grown are used as animal feeds to make meat for man instead of providing food for those who are in need of it. The area of arable land needed to support one person living entirely on meat (as an extreme case), would be sufficient to provide food for ten vegetarians.

AESTHETICS

Few people would continue to eat meat if they visited the slaughterhouses in which the animals are killed. Not many people can fail to be put off by the sight of bloody animal cadavers in butchers' shops.

ETHICS

There is a large movement devoted to animal welfare and the fight against animal exploitation. Many people are deeply concerned about experiments on animals. The slaughter of animals is surely an extreme case of animal exploitation, even if the method is made as painless as possible. There remains the agony of the animal on its way to the slaughterhouse and up to the moment it is killed. The vegans are the only consistent ethical vegetarians, as they rightly argue that by partaking of milk products people promote the killing of bull calves or their sterilization. Many religious people such as Hindus are ethical vegetarians.

ECOLOGY

The loss of animal manure if fewer animals were kept for meat would create an important problem in the ecology, as it would alter the natural environment. But such a loss can be more than made good by proper use of human waste products. They are at present emptied into the sea and rivers, causing pollution. In that way an enormous amount of valuable matter is lost to the land. It could and should be added to the soil. The difficulties and hygienic problems of such an operation can be overcome by proper treatment of sewage by purification plants which convert sewage into non-offensive valuable matter.

The average person does not, however, choose his or her food for ecological and economic reasons. Even aesthetic, ethical and health considerations play a small part for most people Their eating habits are determined by psychological factors, what they fancy and what their families and friends eat and drink. These psychological aspects will now be investigated.

Psychodietetics of natural therapy

The natural diet provides ample choice, which means that you can choose your foods according to your particular taste. A natural therapist must be aware of this personal factor. Effective dietetics is incomplete if the mind is not taken into account. Thus, psychodietetics has to be included within natural therapy.

Psychodietetics, while in itself not a science, does provide for the interrelationship of those sciences that have to do with psychology and nutrition. Sociology, psychology, physiology, home economics, biochemistry, and other special fields where the scientist is inclined to remain segregated in his research laboratory are brought together to give practical information to those who can utilize it.[54]

There is a mutual relationship between the type of food which is consumed and the mind of the consumer: a fault in nutrition adversely affects not only the body but also the mind, and can lead to lassitude, irritability and, in the case of severe deficiencies of such vitamins as nicotinic acid, to insanity. On the other hand, a faulty mental attitude, or emotional illness, can cause you to refuse to eat wholesome food and to neglect your dietetic requirements.

The extent to which natural therapy prevents or corrects physical ailments is obviously valuable from the psychological, as well as from the physical, point of view; for physical ill-health causes mental suffering. If you achieve generally better health through adopting a natural therapy dietetic regime, you will feel better *as a whole person,* which means that your mental condition has benefited from the treatment. As this form of therapy has not been imposed upon you, you will have chosen to change your eating habits in favour of those of natural therapy and you will have the satisfaction of personal achievement if your health improves physically and mentally. Behaving responsibly carries its own reward.

The case for adopting the natural therapy regime is convincing, but people frequently resist convincing arguments and fail to behave in a responsible way. The human mind is not only logical and rational but also emotional and irrational. The natural therapist must be aware of the emotional factors which operate in relation to the implementation of his principles. Psychodietetics have isolated the following factors: hunger, appetite, habit, custom and symbolization.

Hunger

Hunger has been defined as a 'prime drive' in human behaviour. In our affluent society many people hardly know the feeling of hunger, but natural therapy provides them with this elemental sensation. You feel hungry at the beginning of a fast. A reassuring attitude on the part of the therapist is essential to guide you through the stage of hunger, and to prevent you from experiencing any feelings of panic that you are suffering some serious harm by going without food. During a low-calorie diet of fruit and raw vegetables, with some protein such as yoghurt, people who are used to a diet containing more calories also feel hungry. Many of them are too fat; they must learn to bear their hunger if they wish to lose unhealthy and unsightly fat. They 'have learned to turn to food whenever they become anxious or upset'; food for them is 'the short-term panacea for all emotional stress'.[55] A natural therapist can help these patients to give up their compulsion only if he can help them to resolve the emotional conflict which stimulates their voracious hunger, but such treatment requires skilled psychotherapy.

Paradoxically, there is a risk that the compulsive eater may turn totally against food and become a sufferer from *anorexia nervosa.* This is a dangerous condition, as the patients (usually young girls who are afraid of becoming too fat) may starve themselves to death. Unconscious guilt feelings, and the desire for suffering or death, play a part in those whose natural hunger is suppressed. To prescribe a fast or a strict dietetic regime for such patients would be a grave mistake, as the therapist cannot rely on the sound instinct for life which manifests itself in normal hunger.

Appetite

While hunger is an elemental instinctual drive, appetite is just a tendency to eat. Your appetite is stimulated by taste, smell and touch, as well as by the sight of food. Food must be attractive and appetizing. On no account should you feel any revulsion from it, and your individual tastes should be accepted within the framework of natural therapy. This means that you must be helped to replace cravings for unhealthy foods, such as sweets, and pastries made from white flour, by the enjoyment of simple, attractive natural foods, such as salads and fruits. Your appetite is further influenced by emotions; generally, you gain appetite in a relaxed and happy state and soon lose it in a state of tension, anxiety, depression or excitement. Your surroundings often determine the emotional climate, the arousal or suppression of appetite. The therapist must be aware of these facts and try to promote favourable conditions.

Habit

The reform in eating that is advocated by natural therapy is a reform in your habits. Eating sweets, drinking tea and coffee, over-eating in general, are in many cases the result of having fallen into bad habits. Often the fault dates back to childhood. Parents indulge their children by buying them ice-creams, sweets and other unwholesome treats, when they could give them sweet fruits such as dates or grapes instead. Schools feed children on white bread and puddings made from white flour. To break away from such wrongly acquired tastes is difficult if you have become dependent on them. People have to learn to discipline themselves and not rely on unhealthy food and drinks — on endless cups of tea and coffee to stimulate their tired bodies and minds. Once the task has been grappled with, you can experience that change as something exciting. Adopting new and healthy habits is an adventure and not a punishment. It can be exhilarating. This is the attitude which your natural therapist will convey to you.

Custom

We are not only creatures of habit, we are also followers of customs; what other people in our society do becomes our norm. To differ from the crowd is painful because people do not like to be conspicuous.

The natural therapist must consider the social factor, the customs of eating. Children, in particular, suffer if they are not allowed to share in the food at school or at children's parties. Enforcement can cause considerable harm to the children's minds, and the natural therapist may decide to compromise rather than to insist on wholesome food. The case of the adult is easier. He can stand up to friends or relatives, and can explain the reason why customary food is refused. But here also, the strain may be considerable, and it would certainly be wrong if, as a follower of natural therapy, you were to cut yourself off from your social group and become isolated.

Symbolization

Your natural therapist has to be aware of the deeper emotional reasons why people cling to faulty food habits and customs. Eating is pleasurable, and many people resent the discipline of going without certain foods as a deprivation of pleasure. The natural therapist can point to the pleasure of eating wholesome foods, but also, as over-eating is always harmful even though pleasurable at the time, he may have to put to the patient the alternative of the pain of illness to the forgoing of culinary pleasures. People who have been deprived of love and affection, lonely people, take to eating, especially of sweet foods, as a compensation. To them, food stands for comfort, but it can also stand for status. White bread used to be a privilege of the rich, but then it became coveted by the other classes who did not want to be left behind.

Desires for, and refusals of, food can be the expression of deep psychological attitudes. Not to conform, whether to natural therapy or any other school of thought, and to disregard advice, can be an act of aggression or defiance. Food is just one of the means by which it is possible to express such unconscious feelings.

Conclusion

Natural therapists have to meet their patients' needs for food, understood as an expression of body, mind and spirit. The approach is holistic which means as far as the body is concerned, ideally three principles, formulated by Sir Robert McCarrison, a former Director of Research on Nutrition in India, apply: 1. Food should be grown on a healthy soil; 2. Food should be eaten whole; 3. Food should be eaten fresh.[56] As we saw, the science of food technology offends against these principles, as with its fragmentation it fails to do justice to the wholeness of life in the soil, in the food and in people. We also saw how the science of nutrition which considers food to be the supplier of energy for the body-machine equally fails although the scientific approach to such diseases as cancer and heart disease confirmed the validity of the holistic organic approach.

The mind's wholeness differs from the body's. The body functions holistically in a state of integration, whereas the mind's wholeness is achieved by an individual person's resolution of conflicts, mostly of an emotional kind. The preceding section on psychodietetics, dealing with hunger, appetite, habit, custom and symbolization, considered this vital aspect of natural therapy.

The spirit is that part which is concerned with personal freedom, with responsibility, with the acknowledgement and the upholding of values. These aspects of natural therapy have been stressed in this book and their significance for the choice of particular foods has been clarified. Two types of spiritual-ethical nature have been discussed: the first type is related to personal health, to a choice of food which promotes health, accepted as a responsibility. The second type is related to responsibilities for animals, their slaughter and exploitation. Vegans and vegetarians, it was shown, are motivated by such values.

Food with its implications for the body, mind and spirit occupies a central position in natural therapy. Our next task consists in clarifying the relation between your health and the state of your bowel which of course is intimately related to your choice of food.

Chapter 6

Health and your bowel

In order to understand the relationship between health and the bowel, it is necessary to investigate certain mechanical, biochemical and bacterial processes which take place within the bowel.

Mechanics

Adverse mechanical effects arise within the bowel and also affect other parts of the body due to increased pressure from a loaded colon. This condition has already been referred to as a result of the consumption of an excess of refined carbohydrates, characteristic of the saccharine disease, manifest in haemorrhoids, varicose veins in the legs and in the scrotum. Pressure, due to straining with the stool, has the same results, but this time the trouble is caused by lack of fibre in the diet which was stressed earlier as the source of a whole range of diseases.[1] The bulky soft stools, associated with the ingestion of fibre, make such straining unnecessary.

Biochemistry

The relationship between diet and cancer of the large bowel, discussed earlier, has been attributed to a cancer-producing agent in the diet, a 'carcinogen'. Animal experiments have revealed that a fourfold increase in dietary fat raises the level of bile salts in the bowel and that bile acids are responsible for tumour formation in rats.[2] In human beings such biochemical changes, as we saw, are associated also with cancers of the breast and the prostate gland, but the liver and the pancreas are also affected.[3] By comparing a conventional meat diet with a vegetarian diet, the faecal bile content, derived from dietary fat and a source of carcinogens,[4] has been found to be higher in the former, compared with the latter.

Bacteriology

Bacterial processes within the bowel have been referred to as constituting the *bowel flora* which is a manifestation of holistic interaction within the body. The significance of these micro-organisms for a person's health will now be elaborated.

The bowel harbours millions of bacteria of different kinds. They produce enzymes, substances which induce or accelerate chemical reactions in the body. The colonic flora change markedly according to the diet, as evidenced by the measurement of bacterial enzymes. Certain faecal bacteria are far more numerous in meat-eaters than in lacto-vegetarians or vegans. The favourable results of a vegetarian diet, compared with a meat diet, point to the role of the bowel flora in explaining these results.

An antibiotic, taken by mouth, upsets the bowel flora. Such a disturbance is frequently shown by the occurrence of diarrhoea. Antibiotics are prescribed by doctors on a vast scale. Natural therapy makes these prescriptions unnecessary in most cases. (Antibiotics also disturb the bacteriological flora in the mouth and in the vagina, causing a variety of symptoms.)

Natural therapists often recommend yoghurt to normalize the bowel flora. Yoghurt is made by allowing milk to ferment with a culture of certain beneficial germs which include the bacillus acidophylus. Medical scientists have confirmed the benefits of such a recommendation. The colonization of the colon with the lactobacillus is said to reduce the danger of colon cancer.

Finally the intestinal flora have been shown to be related to sex hormones and to the use of the contraceptive pill, taken by many millions of women. It has been demonstrated that by suppressing the intestinal flora with antibiotics, the concentration of the sex hormones in the blood is reduced.[5]

Natural elimination

Moving the bowels is an important function. It has been shown that regular evacuation can be achieved through promoting healthy bowel flora and through a rich fibre content in food. Lack of physical exercise is another factor causing constipation, and a further cause of this common complaint is found in ignoring nature's call; as a result, people become unaware of the fullness of the rectum. This fault often dates back to childhood, when a boy or girl was not trained to visit the toilet before going to school. When the child experienced the urge during lessons, he or she was often too shy to ask to be excused. In such cases, a natural therapist has to re-educate the patient to become aware of the fullness of the rectum and the following yoga exercises against constipation will help.[6]

Exercise 1: (Ghenanda Sambita II, 15, 24; III, 21, 82)
The patient sits with his knees straight. He bends forward and touches his toes with his finger tips, at the same time opening the anus (as if having a motion); on leaning back he contracts the anus. This exercise should be carried out every day for fifteen to twenty minutes, with intervals.

Exercise 2: (Ghenanda Sambita II, 14, 22, 24)
The patient squats in a bath which is partly filled with water; his knees should not touch the floor of the bath and his heels should be pressed against the buttocks. The patient separates the buttocks by pressing his heels apart, and thus opens the anus, at the same time breathing out as deeply as possible. This causes negative pressure on the rectum and a small quantity of water enters. He then closes the anus. He repeats the exercise a few times, thus giving himself an enema and the bowel is then emptied.

Both these exercises, especially the second one, have to be practised for some time before the patient can carry them out well.

Laxatives should be avoided whenever possible, as they tend to lead to more constipation after the stimulation has worn off. Liquid paraffin should not be taken, as it absorbs fat soluble vitamins, thus depriving the body of them. Also, some of the paraffin gets absorbed and collects in the lymph nodes within the abdomen where it can give rise to swellings. 'Isogel' and 'Normacol' are harmless; they induce soft, bulky stools, and the beneficial effect of bran on stool evacuation has been emphasized already.

If the patient's bowels do not move spontaneously, and if neither harmless medicinal aids nor special exercises overcome constipation, natural therapists may resort to the use of suppositories, enemas or colonic irrigation. However, suppositories and enemas should not be given over prolonged periods as they tend to abolish the natural reflex which is nature's call to empty the bowel.

A glycerine suppository or the more drastic 'dulcolax' suppository stimulates the bowel and clears the rectum. An enema can be administered preferably with a gravity douche. The enema consists of lukewarm water or normal saline (1 tablespoon of common salt to one pint of warm water) or of an affusion of herbs such as camomile. Enemas bring about defecation by distending the bowel, but, as with suppositories, people become dependent on them.

A colonic irrigation reaches sections of the lower bowel which are beyond the reach of enemas and suppositories, but the main purpose of irrigation is not just the removal of faeces but the washing out of the bowel. This lavage can improve the tonicity of the bowel wall and thus help to overcome constipation, as the bowel musculature gets stronger. Since natural therapists consider the elimination of toxins to be an important part of their treatment, enemas and colonic irrigations are often combined with the use of eliminative diets, particularly in conjunction with fasts, but the subject is controversial.

One natural therapist considers that any measures which force elimination via the bowels (and also via the skin and the kidneys) during a fast are harmful. Instead, he relies entirely on the inherent healing power within the body which, he claims, causes the bowel to empty itself.[7] Other natural therapists insist that enemas and irrigations form an essential part of the eliminative treatment. High enemas and colonic irrigations are also employed to relieve the spasm in the urinary canal when it is blocked by a stone, and thus facilitate natural passage of the stone. Further benefits from irrigations are claimed in inflammatory conditions of the gall bladder and of the female internal genital organs. In cases of diverticulitis, the contents of the pouches are washed out and the bowel is cleared and encouraged to contract better. The mechanical effects of the large amounts of warm water can also have a beneficial result on the bowel flora. Colonic irrigations must not be used, however, if the anal sphincter is weak, if the patient suffers from painful piles or an anal fissure or a fistula (an abnormal opening of the rectum into the skin), from any other painful anal lesion, from an infection of the lower bowel, or from a growth in the bowel.

The functioning of the bowel is intimately connected with the mind. The natural therapist has to be aware of this relationship and has to realize that constipation and diarrhoea may be the result of emotional disturbances, and that enemas, suppositories and irrigations may have harmful psychological consequences. While elimination is obviously important for general health, bowel-consciousness should be avoided and the idea prevalent in a previous generation that harm is to be expected if evacuation does not occur completely regularly (an idea which led to the abuse of laxatives) must be resisted.

Physiological and psychological factors play a part in all the organs with which the natural therapist is concerned. We shall now discuss the lungs, which stand for the very breath of life.

Chapter 7

The breath of life

A holistic view

The act of breathing has profound significance for the whole body. It is concerned with a supply of oxygen to all tissues and an elimination of carbon dioxide. By breathing in, the volume within the rib cage is increased, the pressure within the small air spaces in the lungs drops causing a suction effect in the large veins, leading to a flow of blood into the right ventricle of the heart. The pump action of the heart is promoted by respiration as more blood is sucked into the lungs, causing the lungs to expand. With expiration the air is pressed out of the lungs bringing blood into the left chamber of the heart. The most important muscle concerned with breathing is the diaphragm. Its movements affect the aorta, the circulation in the liver and spleen, the movements of the contents in the stomach and intestines.

Breathing is rhythmical, governed by a centre in the brain, in response to the amount of carbon dioxide in the blood. There are three phases: inspiration, expiration and pause. When the breathing is calm, the three phases are equal in length. If respiration is rapid, inspiration is shorter than expiration and the pause disappears. When you take a full breath, the diaphragm, the ribs and your spine all take part in the expansion of your lungs. Your abdominal muscles relax during inspiration allowing the abdomen to protrude. When breathing out, these muscles contract and the diaphragm resumes its dome-like shape. The lung volume diminishes.

Faulty breathing consists in insufficient expansion of the rib cage and of the abdominal muscles. The following factors have to be considered in the promotion of proper breathing. Tense muscles have to be relaxed; muscles which are underdeveloped and slack have to be strengthened through exercise. Stiffness of ribs and spine calls for loosening up. Relaxation is important to allow for deep and rhythmical breathing. Deep and full expiration is followed by deep full inspiration. Attention must be paid to all the parts which take part in the respiratory movement, the diaphragm which causes a movement of the abdominal wall, and the ribs which expand when a deep breath is taken. Breathing exercises can be carried out in a sitting position, lying down, standing and walking. The palms can be used to encourage the contraction of the rib cage and of the abdominal wall and they follow the expansion of the lungs by remaining in contact with the ribs and the abdominal wall. The smooth functioning of respiration is of fundamental importance for the functions of the heart and blood vessels.

Exercises for the breathless

People who suffer from breathing trouble, because of chronic bronchitis and damage to the elasticity of lung tissue, benefit from exercises which have been developed at the Brompton Hospital in London, a leading hospital in this field of medicine.[1] Many of these patients suffer from an obstruction of their airways. If they are told to force the air out of their lungs, this obstruction gets worse. It is better to encourage relaxation which promotes breathing activity.

As it is important for these patients to make full use of their diaphragms, diaphragmatic breathing is taught. Figures 1 and 2 illustrate this exercise.

The explanations are as follows:

Figure 1   The best position is a half-lying position in a comfortable chair, with the back well supported. The patient places his hands on the lower end of his rib cage, is told to relax and to breathe out gently, allowing his upper abdomen and the rib margins in front to sink down and in, without contracting the abdominal muscles. Then he is told to breathe in gently and to 'feel the air coming around his waist[2] without using any force. This exercise can be used during attacks of breathlessness with good effect.

Figure 2   This method mobilizes the lower ribs. The patient's palm is placed on the lower ribs on a line which runs down from the armpit. He is told to breathe out and to feel his lower ribs sinking in and down. When he breathes in, he should be instructed to expand his lower ribs

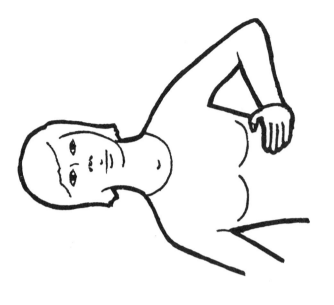

Figure 2
Localized basal expansion

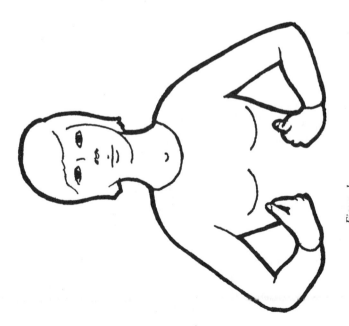

Figure 1
Diaphragmatic breathing

against the firm pressure of his hands, trying to direct the incoming air to the base of this lung. After six breaths, the same procedure is repeated on the other side. With regular practice the pattern of breathing can often be improved.

As relaxation is essential when breathing is laboured, a number of positions are assumed which all encourage relaxation.

Figure 3   The patient is sitting on a chair, leaning over a table on which two or three pillows are placed, the patient leaning forward against them, able to relax.

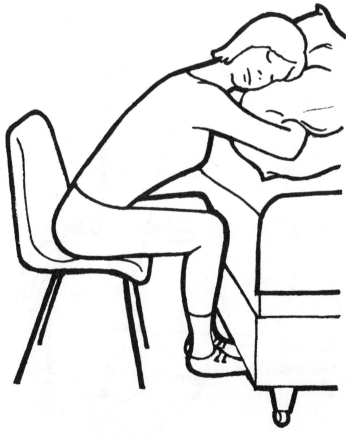

Figure 3
Relaxation position
(forward leaning sitting)

Figure 4 A useful position to encourage relaxation, allowing the shoulders to drop, instead of being raised which people in states of breathing trouble are inclined to do.

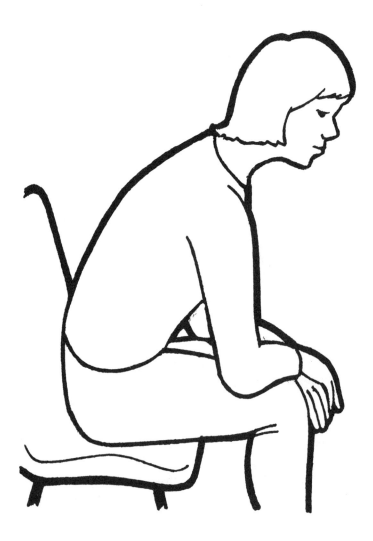

Figure 4
Relaxation position
(relaxed sitting)

Figure 5   Breathless people may be unable to lie down or to sit up. They prefer standing. They should be encouraged to lean forward on some available object and to relax at the same time.

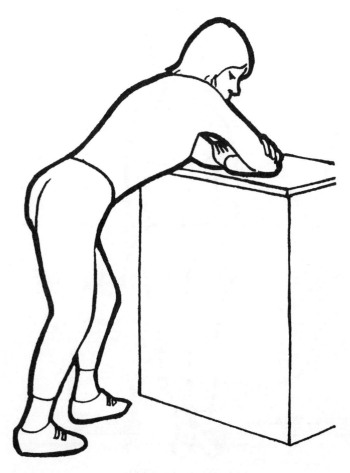

Figure 5
Relaxation position
(forward leaning
standing)

Figure 6 A person who is distressed by breathlessness may find it easier when standing up leaning his back against a wall, his feet slightly away from the wall, his pelvis resting against it. Shoulders and arms should be relaxed.

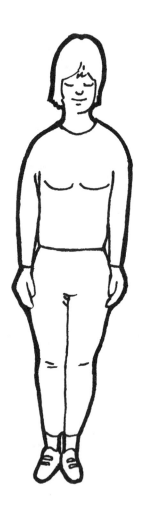

Figure 6
Relaxation position
(relaxed standing)

If bronchial secretions accumulate within the bronchial tubes, it may be necessary to allow them to drain away rather than be coughed up. To achieve this drainage, the patient should lie on his side in a sloping position with his head lower than his pelvis. Figure 7 illustrates this. It shows the patient lying on a six-inch-thick pile of newspapers or magazines, tied together, with two pillows on top of them. The patient has to practise his breathing exercises in this position to loosen the secretions and to cough at intervals with five to ten minutes to be spent on either side.

As an alternative, the foot of the bed can be raised 12-18 inches from the ground, but this is often impractical at home.

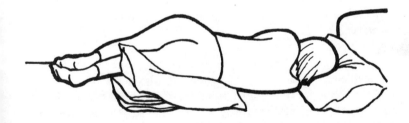

Figure 7
Postural drainage
at home

Chapter 8

Natural stimulation and your skin

Skin - not just a body envelope

In order to appreciate the significance of the natural treatment of the skin, we must understand what role this organ plays in the maintenance of health. Although essential as the 'body envelope' - a guard against the outer world - the skin also has its own vital functions, which are integrated with those of the whole organism. In addition, the skin is important for mental well-being. A healthy skin is beautiful and attractive, and an unhealthy skin is ugly; thus the condition of the skin can make a person self-confident or insecure. Many people who have skin blemishes feel self-conscious, embarrassed and depressed on account of their appearance, and in such cases natural therapy helps to provide not only better physical health but also a desperately needed mental uplift.

The functions of the skin point to the vital role of this organ for the body as a whole. The skin protects the body against mechanical, thermal, electrical and chemical injuries. It helps in the maintenance of body temperature, stores large quantities of water and salts, resists the invasion of germs, and absorbs gases and fatty substances. The skin is richly supplied with blood vessels. The nerves in the skin provide us with information received through touch, including a whole range of experiences including voluptuous sensations, itching, burning, and various types of pain. The sebaceous glands in the skin secrete a greasy substance which keeps the skin supple, and the sweat glands are of particular importance, since toxins are eliminated in perspiration.

Surface elimination

The significance of sweating for general health has been emphasized in a paper by Dr St John Lyburn. He maintains that 'to sweat is a function as essential for human existence as eating, sleeping and defecation. A normal healthy adult sweats nearly a pint a day which evaporates, leaving a layer of minute waste products on the surface of the skin.' The total area of sweat glands is related to the total area of skin: 'the skin is the largest organ of the body. It covers an area between sixteen and twenty square feet, and each of us has between four and five million active sweat glands.' If they were put together they would 'form an opening as large as the mouth'.[1]

Heat treatment
Dry heat, applied to the whole body - the Sauna

The sauna is a dry hot-air bath which includes jets of moist air introduced for brief periods. The exposure to heat of 100-200°F (38°-94°C) lasts for ten minutes and is followed by an exposure to cool air or to cold water for fifteen minutes, and then by a rest for a further fifteen minutes. In Finland, the country of its origin, the sauna is a national institution. It is visited at least once a week for cleansing purposes, and after strenuous exercise it is part of training for sportsmen. The sauna has become popular in other countries, and its effects on the body have been closely studied. The change from heat to cold has beneficial effects on the heart, as it tends to regulate blood pressure. Physical fitness is increased in a way which is not achieved by the usual forms of physical training. Through perspiration, considerable amounts of sodium, and smaller quantities of potassium are excreted. This is important with regard to the alkali/acid balance in the body. (As sodium and potassium are factors which increase the alkali component in the blood, people who lose these substances in their sweat have to replace them by taking such alkaline foods as fruit and vegetables, including salad. The proportionate loss of potassium is smaller than that of sodium, which has therapeutic significance, as sodium - the alkaline component of common salt - is often present in excessive amounts in the body.)[2]

The study was concerned only with changes occurring in healthy young people, and its authors did not examine any sick persons. Their results point to the importance of this form of heat for attaining and retaining fitness, but as no precautions are taken with regard to keeping the head cool, the sauna is a drastic form of treatment for people who are not fit, although it has its uses. For instance, rheumatologists have reported beneficial effects: weekly sauna treatments are apparently of considerable help to patients suffering from rheumatoid arthritis; they tend to prevent fresh attacks of the disease.[3]

Attention has, however, been drawn to the dangers of this form of heat application. A preliminary investigation by the US Federal Trade Commission found that the rise in body temperature, blood pressure and pulse rate in the sauna constitutes a risk to elderly people and to sufferers from diabetes, heart disease and high blood pressure. There is further danger if steam baths or sauna baths are taken within an hour after eating or while under the influence of alcohol or the following drugs: anticoagulants, antihistamines, vasoconstrictors, vasodilators, stimulants, narcotics, tranquillizers. The duration of the sauna must be strictly limited, and care taken to make sure that people do not exceed the time allowed.[4]

The effects of the sauna on people's health has recently been re-examined by two Finnish doctors. Their findings were reported in the *British Medical Journal.*[5]

The Sauna Society of Finland 'recommends that the temperature at the level of the face should be 80-90°C and the humidity 50-60 g of water vapour for each cubic metre. The stay in the hot room is normally limited to about 10 minutes at a time, and three exposures to the hot room are usual.' These figures were not always found, as the temperature varied from 43°C to 120°C and the humidity from 3 per cent to 50 per cent. Some people spent up to several hours in the sauna.

Effects on the heart were found to include an increase of the pulse rate to 100-160 beats per minute, the blood vessels in the skin dilated and the blood output of the heart was increased. There were varying effects on the blood pressure. The immersion in cold water reverses the effects of the heat. Sometimes the blood pressure goes up considerably as the result of exposure to cold. During a sauna at least 0.5 kg of sweat may be lost.

Amongst the Finns, the sauna has not been found to have any harmful effects on the heart, even in people who suffer from heart disease, 'as long as exposure is reasonable and cooling off moderate'. But the article warns that 'those with heart disease, the elderly and novices should adopt a gentle approach': only five minutes in the hot room at first. It advises people who are feverish, who have recently lost body fluids, have taken strenuous exercise, or who are unable to perspire, not to use the sauna. Spending too long in the hot room is dangerous. The effect on the psyche, tranquillity, is confirmed[6]

Local application of heat

Apart from applying heat to the whole skin, a natural therapist can selectively deal with parts of the body. Hot water can be applied as fomentations, consisting of one layer of lint wrung out in hot water, covered with oil-silk or plastic material, which is in turn covered with cotton wool. In this way heat is kept in, and the lint can be renewed every few hours. Hot fomentations are very useful in the treatment of contaminated wounds (for instance abrasions), since this method removes grit and pus, and a clean healing surface is obtained.

As another local application, steam from a disconnected kettle can be directed by means of a funnel on to inflamed parts such as the nose or the anus, for the relief of pain and, in the case of piles, for the relief of congestion. Care must be taken to prevent scalding.

A hot arm bath is useful in angina pectoris, which is caused by narrowing of the arteries within the heart muscle. When the arteries in the arm are relaxed, the blood supply to the heart improves through reflex action.

Dry heat and moist heat (as in hot compresses), applied to the abdomen, relieve pain arising from intestinal colic and, applied to the loins, help in cases of renal pain due, for instance, to stone formation.

Many painful conditions, especially sprains and bruises, respond to alternative applications of first hot (five minutes) and then cold (half a minute) treatments.

Cold treatment

A warm skin can be the result of an application of cold air or cold water; this type of 'hyperaemia' of increased blood supply, is due to the body responding to the stimulus of coldness by producing its own heat. The natural therapist can make full use of this natural response, but it is important to discover how an individual's skin will react to the cold stimulus.

In order to assess this response, a writer working at the Spa Wörishofen in Germany, where cold-water treatment is carried out extensively, classified his patients according to constitutional types. The 'athletic' person can stand only infrequent, fairly strong applications of cold; the fat, short person or 'pyknic' can tolerate cold applications (especially cold compresses) well, and quite drastic treatment can be given. The slenderly built 'asthenic' needs warmth. In this last case, only a small area of skin should be exposed to the cold and only for a short time. The bloated, 'lymphatic' type also lacks resistance to cold, although resistance can be raised by carefully graded cold applications.

Apart from this classification according to physical types, different-iation has also been made according to psychological make-up. The circulation of the neurasthenic, emotionally weak person, is easily upset by cold, and hence great care is needed. The melancholic is slow to react and in this case a strong stimulus is needed in order to achieve any result. The sanguine type, on the other hand, responds quickly and may even ask for a strong stimulus, but caution is called for here, as the patient may be rash in his judgement and may over-estimate his physical stamina. The choleric, irascible type must learn to relax and, in this case, only lukewarm water is suitable. Generally speaking, it has been found that skin which is dry and hot responds well to repeated cold sponging, whereas a moist skin gives a better response to a wet compress.

In cases of heart failure and high blood pressure, drastic cold-water treatment should be avoided but, on the other hand, such patients benefit when made to perspire, as congestion is relieved through perspiration.[7]

The texture, colour and temperature of the skin give guidance to the natural therapist. A very dry skin lacks sweat glands, and therefore such a patient cannot bear heat. Neither will the person who perspires heavily be a suitable subject for intensive cold water treatment, as he is frequently a neurasthenic who shows poor response. Vinzenz Priessnitz, a peasant, who was one of the pioneers of water treatment, chose the stimulus of coldness according to the patient's immediate response to cold water. Blanching pointed to a lack of response, whilst a glowing skin indicated suitability.

Apart from these general responses, cold-water applications have an effect on the following organs: when applied to the arms or the left side of the chest, they slow the heart-beat but increase the output of blood from the heart. They have a soothing effect on the thyroid gland, stimulate bowel movement, and deepen breathing. Cold foot-baths increase kidney activity, tend to calm the patient and thus can promote sleep; they also relieve congestion of the head by drawing blood away from it. Cold water has an effect on the nerves which supply the blood vessels, and the result is an initial rise of blood pressure which is followed by a fall, while the tone of the vessel wall can be improved by the cold stimulus. When the stimulus has been too drastic, the patient may complain of palpitation, congestion of the head, giddiness and shortness of breath.

Father Kneipp's water cure
Exercise
Father Kneipp was a pioneer of cold-water treatment. His recommendations included walking barefoot in wet grass for fifteen to forty-five minutes a day, on wet stones for three to fifteen minutes, in recently fallen snow for three to fifteen minutes, or in cold water (which should first reach to the ankle and later to the knee) for one to six minutes. After such exercise, the patient immediately puts on dry socks and shoes. These instructions illustrate the grading of the cold-water stimulus; for in each case it must be adjusted to the person's ability to respond, and any drastic, harmful measure is avoided - a principle also valid when using the cold compress.

Compress
The cold compress consists of a piece of linen wrung out in cold water, covered by several layers of dry wool. The whole compress is held together by large safety pins. The grading of the stimulus is achieved by varying the thickness of the moist layer, and also the area of the body in contact with the compress. Kneipp distinguished between the 'lower compress' which reaches from the armpits to the hips, and the 'upper compress' which extends from the nape of the neck to the end of the spine. In addition, he used compresses for the chest, the neck, the hands, the arms, the feet, the calves, the whole leg and the sacral region.

For a good response, the following conditions must be fulfilled: the patient must feel warm before and after the application of the compress (which is a sign that his body has responded to the water stimulus). To obtain a favourable response, the linen must envelop the particular part of the body tightly, and the woollen layers must overlap the linen. If the compress covers the chest, back or abdomen, the whole body must be kept warm by blankets, and the patient's arms must be beneath the covers. A hot bath taken before the application of a cold compress, or hot-water bottles given while the patient is in the compress, can be used to help him to get warm and he can also be given sips of hot fluids. With the feeling of warmth, perspiration sets in.

The compress is left in position until the perspiration has stopped, then the linen is removed and the patient is left in the woollen layers - for instance, wrapped in a blanket (a turkish towel can be interposed between the linen and the wool to absorb the perspiration). At this stage, many patients start to sweat again, but in a milder form. When the patient has finally ceased to perspire, the rest of the compress is removed and his whole skin is sponged with cold water, and dried. Even if there is no visible perspiration, the compress is effective and can be left on, provided the patient feels warm. Vinegar and herbs can be added to the water in which the linen is wrung out. If the patient has not reacted with a feeling of warmth within ten minutes, the compress must be removed.

The cold-water compress causes perspiration and helps to eliminate toxic substances, especially when it covers the trunk. The particular effects on individual organs, quoted from St John Lyburn's paper, give further indications for the use of the cold compress. In cases of fever, perspiration is present anyway, and the compress is easily warmed up (except when the patient complains of shivering). It assists in the elimination of toxins during a feverish illness. A combination of different compresses is frequently called for. For instance, in the case of tonsillitis, a compress around the neck can help the local inflammatory process, while a waist compress can promote elimination of toxins. A cold compress on the forehead can relieve the headache which accompanies the fever. Inflammation of veins in the leg (phlebitis) is treated with a leg compress: a thin stocking wrung out in cold water, covered by a dry thick (woollen) stocking.

The technique of applying a cold compress to the body from the neck downwards and one covering the chest and abdomen will now be illustrated and the method of covering the patient to avoid getting cold will be shown in separate pictures.

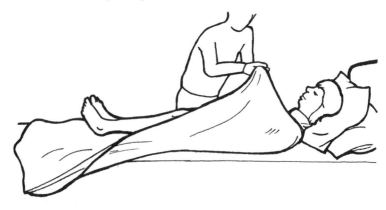

*Figure 1: Cold compress covering body
from neck downwards.*

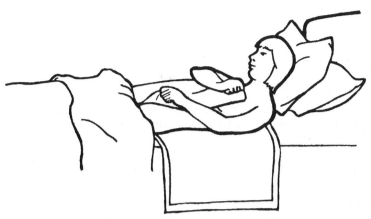

Figure 2: Cold compress covering chest and abdomen.

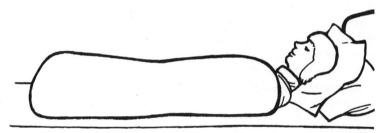

Figure 3: Correct: patient covered up carefully, arms under the blanket. Neck protected by linen against contact with blanket.

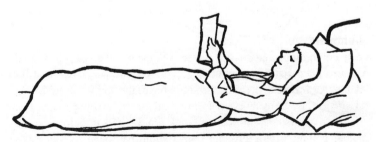

Figure 4: Incorrect: arms outside blanket so patient is not kept warm.

Baths

Father Kneipp gave detailed prescriptions for various forms of baths. Cold foot-baths, for example, lasting one to three minutes, draw blood away from the head and chest and are recommended to relieve fatigue and sleeplessness. They can be combined with hot foot-baths to which hay flower, oat straw or malt husks may be added.

The stimulus of the cold bath can be varied according to the area of the skin immersed. The most drastic form is the full cold bath in which the patient may stay from half a minute to three minutes. Kneipp considered that this kind of bath should not be taken more often than three times a week. Partial baths, reaching to the calves, knees, thighs, or stomach are less drastic than full baths and, for inflammatory conditions especially, Kneipp advised head, eye and other localized baths.

Affusions

An affusion consists of a shower of cold water which can be applied from a watering can or a hose. The water should flow down the body, enveloping the skin and graduations are again achieved by varying the area of the body, the time of treatment and the temperature of the water.

Damp and wet sheets and dry clothes put on wet skin

In swathing, dry linen, flannel or wool is applied to different parts of the body, which have previously been sponged with cold water. The swathing is kept in position for not longer than 30 minutes and is more effective when combined with hot water. In addition, Kneipp applied wet, coarse linen sheets of various sizes directly to the skin, a more drastic treatment than the cold compress. He also advised patients to wash their bodies with cold water but not to dry the skin, as the evaporation of the water which occurs while the patient dresses in warm clothes and stays in a warm room, has an invigorating effect.[8]

Combinations in hydrotherapy

When combining cold or hot water treatments, the natural therapist considers the patient's constitution and the seriousness of his condition. He may, for instance, order a cold sponging of the upper part of the body on rising, followed by a rest in a warm bed for half an hour, while in the evening the patient should take a quick, cold sitz bath before retiring. Another patient with a stronger constitution may benefit from a cold, all-over sponge each morning and a full body compress each night.

Special forms of water treatment have been devised for patients suffering from arthritis and phlebitis. Here, the stimulus is directed to the arms and legs, using lukewarm or cold water for partial immersion of the limbs and also in the form of a jet of water. As a result, the circulation is improved and the patient experiences warmth, while the joints and veins benefit from the improved circulation. The whole organism gains greater resistance to infections through the training of the circulatory system.[9]

Patients suffering from high blood pressure can also be helped by hydrotherapy. Using one method, the arms, feet and lower half of the trunk are immersed in cold water for 30 minutes every day, while the temperature is raised slowly from 37° to 42°C (98.6°F to 107.6°F). The patient then rests in bed for one to two hours, parts of his body having been covered with cold compresses. This regime has been combined with air baths, walking, gymnastics, breathing exercises, and other forms of physical exercise. The diet consists of wholemeal bread, milk or buttermilk, and vegetables and fruit. The blood pressure falls in a high proportion of cases.[10]

Air treatment

To the natural therapist, air is important not only as the source of the oxygen which we inhale, but also as a stimulus that affects the skin. Air is trapped in the clothes you wear, and so helps to conserve the temperature of your body. In addition, the natural therapist considers the effects which air around the body surface has on the activity of sweat glands. Clothes should be porous to allow you to perspire; cotton underwear fulfils this function better than nylon, while wool soaks up perspiration and is liable to produce excessive heat, leading to undue sweating. Such over-heating of the body is followed by a chilling evaporation of the sweat and can lower the body's resistance to infection. A woollen scarf worn tightly around the neck invites such undesirable consequences.

The ground plays an important part; if, for instance, it consists of white sand, it reflects the rays of the sun and does not absorb as much warmth as dark humus ground which retains heat well. If the ground is uneven, the force of air currents is broken. Another important factor is the degree of moisture which evaporates from the ground; this, together with the air temperature, affects the functions of the skin.

The metabolism of plants is another factor; for they give out oxygen and carbon dioxide, to which are added any gaseous emanations from the soil. A further consideration is the degree of humidity. Dry, cold air is stimulating; it invigorates by increasing the metabolic rate. Whereas intense moist heat encourages perspiration, warm moist air has the opposite effect, especially if there is no wind; it interferes with perspiration and thus with the excretion of toxic substances from the skin. A sultry atmosphere tends to hinder the production of substances which make the body immune to disease. As a result, people feel lethargic and depressed and lack appetite.[11]

The natural therapist welcomes a change from cold to warm, and from dry to moist, as such alterations also act as stimuli (apart from exposure to dry, cold air). These stimuli are missed by people who live in even temperatures, especially if their homes are air-conditioned. Frequently, the recommendation is to wear fewer layers of clothing.

To sum up: the three elements, temperature, wind and moisture, with their variations, determine the effects which air has on the skin. These effects are combined in the air bath.

The air bath

People vary in their ability to stand up to cold, and the natural therapist must adapt air baths (like all other forms of natural treatment) to the individual patient's capacity to respond. He must also keep in mind that the air bath not only affects the patient's skin, but also influences the lungs, since the temperature, moisture and degree of purity of the air modify the depth of breathing and the secretion from the mucus-forming glands in the bronchial tree. At the beginning patients' bodies should be only partly exposed to cool air; later the whole body should be uncovered. Air baths can be given in bed; the room may be heated, and the duration of the air bath must be adjusted to the patient's condition. Taken out-of-doors, air baths are best combined with exercises or with the playing of games.

With regard to individual diseases, there are no strict guidelines for the natural therapist; for, as I have shown, he is mainly concerned with the individual person's reaction to a natural stimulus. He must, however, also consider the diagnostic classification, which is fundamental in scientific medicine. Air baths with their accompanying effects on the lungs, are helpful in feverish diseases. In cases of bronchitis, the lungs benefit from an improved function of the skin, but the effect of the temperature and moisture of the air needs careful assessment. Some people's coughs get worse when they inhale cool air, others are helped. Since the skin is an excretory organ it acts in co-operation with the kidneys, and air baths are recommended in chronic nephritis. There is a further relationship between the skin and the lining of the joints; hence air baths are helpful in the various forms of arthritis. These are a few examples; the list is far from being complete. Air treatment is often combined with, and is itself an essential part of, sun treatment.

Sun treatment

When prescribing sun treatment, the natural therapist is guided by the intensity of the response which is to be expected. The first or mildest degree consists in a sensation of warmth which is due to an increase of blood flow. At the same time the sebaceous and sweat glands are stimulated, but perspiration is visible only if the air is humid. Tanning occurs according to the person's ability to produce pigment. After a longer exposure the second degree of response is characterized by slight redness which is followed in the course of the next few days by tanning, and here we are dealing with a mild form of inflammation of the skin. The third degree, when the patient has been too long in the sun, consists of more intense inflammation which can go on to blister formation, accompanied by general malaise and sometimes shock and fever. A light skin is much more likely to be burnt than a dark one, and fair-skinned people are also sensitive to exposure to wind which reduces their tolerance to sunshine.[12] Whereas an immediate adverse effect is sunburn, the prime danger of over-exposure to the sun is in the possible formation of skin cancer. A recent increase in cases of malignant melanoma, the most dangerous skin tumour, has been attributed to injudicious exposure to the sun.

The power of the sun is greater during the morning, before it has reached its zenith and it is, of course, stronger during the summer months than during the rest of the year. When the sun is very hot, the leaves of a tree provide very good protection against an overdose, but, in any case, the head must be shaded. Reflections from the ground and from the sea intensify the effects of sun on the skin. At high altitudes the force is increased; if the ground is snow-covered, the reflection is intensified; hence exposure must be shorter. Patients can stand sun-treatment better when moving about than when resting; therefore it is a good plan to combine heliotherapy with gymnastics and games. Over-heating has to be avoided (as otherwise there is a danger of sunstroke); cold-water applications are helpful here. On the other hand, chilling is a danger when there is a cold wind, and people may have to cover parts of their bodies.

Sunlight treatment played a most important part in the years before the discovery of the antibiotic drugs which have a specific effect on tubercular infections of bones, joints, internal organs (kidneys and peritoneum, for instance), and the skin. These conditions responded dramatically to sunlight. The pioneer of this treatment was A. Rollier, working in Switzerland. Although there is no further need for his sunlight cure for 'surgical' tuberculosis, the natural therapist of today can draw inspiration from the changes in people's health which Rollier and his associates achieved; for patients whose bodies had become emaciated through a tubercular infection were transformed into well-nourished, strong people. The sun cured not only their tuberculosis, but brought about excellent general health.

Apart from stimulating the blood vessels and glands of the skin, the sun stimulates the underlying muscles. Other organs also benefit, partly because vasodilation in the skin leads to a reduction in congestion elsewhere. The blood supply to the organ which is affected by disease is of importance, for a highly vascular tissue (lungs, peritoneum) reacts more violently than a less vascular structure (e.g. the lining of a knee joint).[13] Rollier further stressed effects on the nervous system, effects starting from the nerve-endings in the skin and continuing by reflex action to other parts of the body, and generally stimulating the metabolism. The ultraviolet rays of the sun also have a bactericidal action; hence sunlight acts as an aseptic and antiseptic treatment for wounds.

Ultraviolet light enables the body to produce vitamin D. Research indicates that the short-wavelength (ultraviolet) radiations of the sun spectrum, not absorbed by the skin, are mostly absorbed by the blood, whereas only 20 per cent of the red and yellow rays and only one per cent of the blue and violet rays pass through the skin.[14]

Whether the sun has a direct effect on the formation of blood corpuscles or whether the effect is indirect, beneficial results in cases of anaemia are well-known. The rays of the sun also lead to absorption of fluid (exudates) in joint cavities, in the peritoneum, and in the pleural cavity. Abscesses heal, repair takes place in previously damaged structures such as joints and bones, and the patient loses his pain. Under the influence of the sun, body temperature rises and, if the treatment is too drastic, nervous excitement and sleeplessness may ensue.

Apart from these physiological effects, the sun affects the mind. People enjoy sunbathing and its bracing effect combined with cool air; under this treatment children lose their fretfulness, and both children and adults feel cheerful. Rollier maintained that sun-bathing is 'the finest stimulus'.[15]

Rollier recommended the following technique for sun baths: they are given three times a day and are graded. On the first day, only the feet are exposed, for five minutes; on the second day, the legs are in the sun for five minutes, and the feet for ten; on the third day, the thighs are included for five minutes; the legs now receive ten and the feet fifteen minutes sunshine. As further areas are uncovered gradually, the whole body up to the neck benefits from the sun. The patient's disease, his general health, and his ability to produce pigment form the guidelines.

Cases of pulmonary tuberculosis, of peritonitis and of heart disease must be treated with particular caution.

(When artificial sunlight with an ultraviolet mercury lamp is used, Rollier's technique can be followed, but the gradual exposure is not essential.) Many patients can stand the sun on the whole body from the beginning of the treatment, provided the sun is not too hot and the head is shaded.

The treatment can be given at low altitudes, and the fact that the sky is overcast does not exclude radiation effects. However, the treatment at low altitudes has certain disadvantages; for, when there is a high degree of humidity, the heat in the summer months is more depressing than in higher regions, and seasonal variations with fewer sunny days have to be accepted. On the other hand, there is the advantage that the patient's body does not have to adapt itself to drastic changes, and this factor is particularly important in cases of diseases of the kidneys and heart and in excitable people. Psychological benefits do not depend on the altitude.[16]

Keeping in mind that debilitating diseases, especially tuberculosis of the lungs and heart disease, are as a rule not suitable for sun treatment (as the necessary response cannot be expected), heliotherapy remains a valuable asset to the natural therapist. Skin conditions such as some vulgaris and psoriasis benefit from the sun, and some cases of neuritis including sciatica also react favourably. Apart from such local effects, the natural therapist values heliotherapy for its general tendency to invigorate.

Chapter 9

Posture, exercise and relaxation

Your spine

The natural therapist not only instructs you about diet, about various applications to the skin, and about how to pay proper attention to breathing and the health of the bowels; he also teaches you how to use your body from a mechanical point of view. This re-education is of vital importance for the person who has 'forgotten' the correct way to stand, walk and relax. Matthias Alexander was a pioneer in this field; his pupil, Charles A. Neill, summarized his teachings in a booklet entitled *Poise and Relaxation.*[1] Neill pointed out that 'more and more people today suffer from poor posture', a factor which leads to faulty co-ordination of movement, and hence to tension. He cited a number of factors which are responsible for this state: anxiety, imitation of parents' habits, illness, and injuries. Whatever initially causes wrong posture, a habit is formed which persists, and he reminded us of some of the consequences: 'A wrong way of standing can lead to aching legs and backache, so too can bad habits in sitting, walking and lifting.' Apart from the direct effects upon our muscles, there are more remote effects on our general health, for instance, leading to faulty breathing and strain.

Good posture is fundamental and consists in the correct relationship of the vertebrae and the head. It gives us poise and is essential for physical attractiveness. The following two drawings help us to understand the mechanics, and Neill's comments provide an excellent explanation:

1 'The spine is not straight and should not be straightened. The curves of the spine are for your protection.

2 'The spine is the core of your body, not just something inserted at the back. Only in the upper part of the back do the bones come away from

the middle line. It may help if you think of the spine as a coiled spring, which should assume its full length - neither compressed, nor stretched, but released.

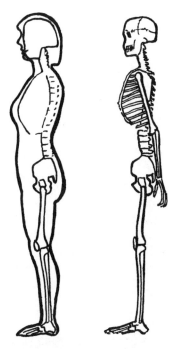

Your spine is a series of curves, all of them important and all of them affecting posture at every point in your body.

3   'The chest is made of curved bones - ribs - which move on the twelve spinal bones of the upper back. An over-curved or over-straight spine will restrict your rib movements and therefore your breathing.

4   'In the lower back the bones are very large and strong, with good thick pads of gristle between as shock absorbers. Yet it is here that most "disk" troubles occur. This is because so many people bend the spine when stooping and lifting, rather than bending the big hip and knee joints. If this area of your spine is too hollow, or curved inwards, your abdomen will protrude. If you flatten your spine you will have backache. The curve must be just right.

5   'Note the big powerful joints of the hips. Feel them on your own body. They are much lower down than most people imagine. Bend from there, also bending your knees, instead of curving your back.

6 'Looking at the skeleton ⟦ from the front ⟧, you will see that the thigh bones are not straight. They curve inward. This is especially so in a woman, since the woman's pelvis is wider. Many people, because of this, unconsciously press the knees apart because they feel knock-kneed. This is wrong and also leads to strain.

7 'The shoulder girdle consists of the collar-bones and the shoulder-blades. They join the rest of the skeleton at the top of the chest. Keep the upper part of your back right and you will not need to bother much about your shoulders - they will fall into their correct place without effort on your part.

'The position of the bones affects the muscles and ligaments attached to them. The postural muscles hold the body up against gravity.'

Neill applied knowledge of anatomical principles to teach correct standing, sitting and walking.

Standing, sitting and walking
Standing
Three pictures serve as illustrations: two faulty extremes which he termed 'too slumped' and 'too braced', and one which is 'just right'. In the slumped position, the muscles do little work and there is strain on the ligaments that hold the bones together, the curves of the spine are exaggerated, the pelvis is tilted forward, and the abdomen is sagging. The lower part of the back is too hollow, causing strain and fatigue.

In the second faulty position, the muscles are too contracted. The bracing of the shoulders backwards leads to tension in the muscles of the shoulder girdle, which results in stiffness and pain. The pushing out of the chest prevents full rib movement and this fault restricts breathing. The holding in of the stomach interferes with the abdominal part of respiration. The 'tucking-in of the tail' makes for tension in buttocks and thighs, going down to the feet.

You are advised to check the correctness of your posture by looking into a long mirror, or even two mirrors. In this way, you can train yourself to adopt the right stance. The feet should be in line, just slightly off parallel. The body's weight is spread evenly over the whole surface of both feet (hence no high heels). The feet are soft and relaxed, the toes uncurled and not gripping the floor. The legs are straight, but not braced back. The whole body gently expands, the spine is straightened, the arms hang easily, the ribs move with the abdomen during rhythmical breathing. All the joints are free, and the whole body feels light. After correct posture has been mastered in the standing position, you can learn how to sit correctly.

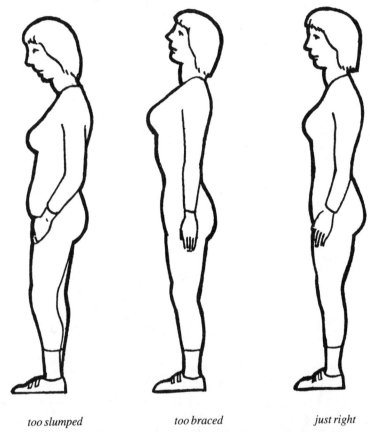

too slumped   *too braced*   *just right*

Sitting

In sitting, as in standing, slumping must be avoided. The spine should be straight without being stretched, the shoulders should be neither braced nor drooping, making breathing effortless. The feet should be on the floor, slightly apart so that there is no tension in them or in the calves, thighs or buttocks, and the hands should rest lightly on the thighs. Illustrations of a woman sitting in a wooden chair and of another in an armchair show the faults of posture which may be encouraged by a faulty armchair; the other pictures demonstrate the correct way to sit.

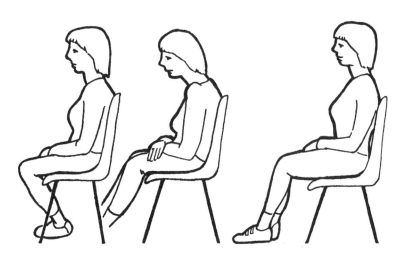

wrong   *wrong again*   *right*

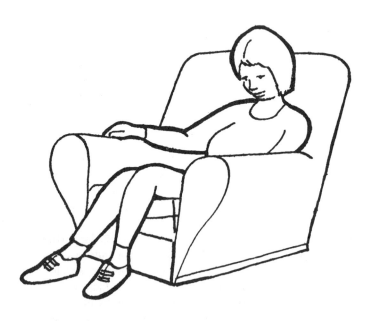

wrong

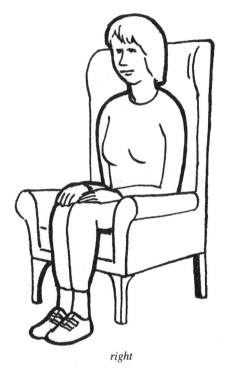

right

A firm high-backed chair is preferable.

Walking

The upright posture, which keeps the body in correct alignment while standing and sitting, should be maintained when walking. Neill stressed the need to balance the head, the neck muscles, and the spine, with the head held level, the eyes looking straight ahead, and the chin neither tucked in nor jutting out. The body should be upright but not braced, and the pelvis should not be too far forward, as such a tilt upsets the proper balance, causing backache. Any swaying from side to side and bobbing up and down should be avoided. When walking with the right posture, a person will be aware of the free movement of hips, knees and ankles.[2]

Apart from following Matthias Alexander's system, the natural therapist encourages his patient to carry out exercises to keep the body supple.

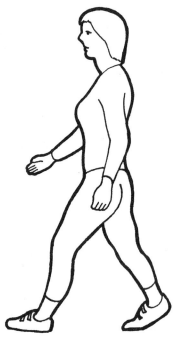

A system of exercises

The system which has been selected aims at keeping healthy people supple and at enabling the sick to regain mobility and thus improve their general health. Thirteen exercises have been compiled by Kenneth Crutchfield and form part of a wider discussion on natural therapy in the home. He recommends that the exercises should be performed slowly at first, and then more quickly, as the person gains strength. They 'are calculated to put the body through all its normal actions',[3] and are carried out while standing, lying, crouching on hands and knees and, again, while standing.

Standing
Exercise 1
Position yourself as in the figure.
(a) Rotate your head from your right shoulder down and forward to the left shoulder, then up and back to the first position. Then reverse the movement. Repeat sequence twelve times.
(b) Rock your head back and forth and from side to side and turn your head fully from side to side. All these movements can be repeated twelve times.

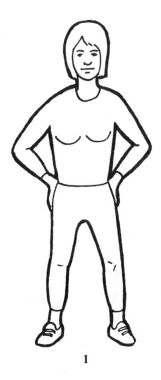

1

Exercise   2
(a) Standing with feet apart swing one arm (other arm on hip) from shoulder high down across your chest then upwards passing your face making a circle back to the original position. Repeat twelve times. Also repeat with other arm.
(b) With one arm back in line with your side (the other on your hip) swing forwards, upwards and back, making a complete circle. Repeat twelve times. Repeat with other arm.
(c) Repeat exercise with both arms together.

Exercise   3
(a) Bend your trunk from the hips (do not strain beyond your capacity), then move your trunk down to the right, across to the left and back to the original standing position repeating this six times.

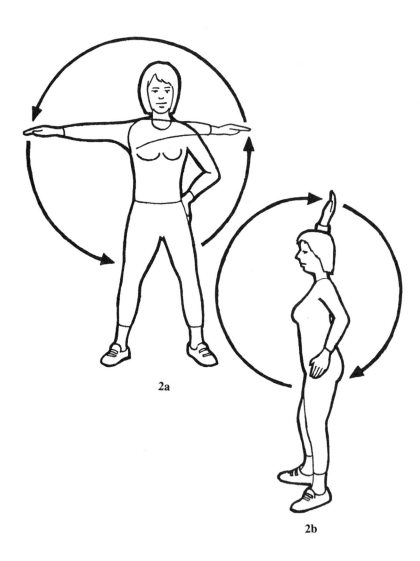

2a

2b

(b) Then move your trunk forwards and rotate it to the right, backwards, across to the left and forward again. Reverse the direction and repeat up to twelve times. To increase the benefit of this exercise, carry out the movements with arms raised above your head.

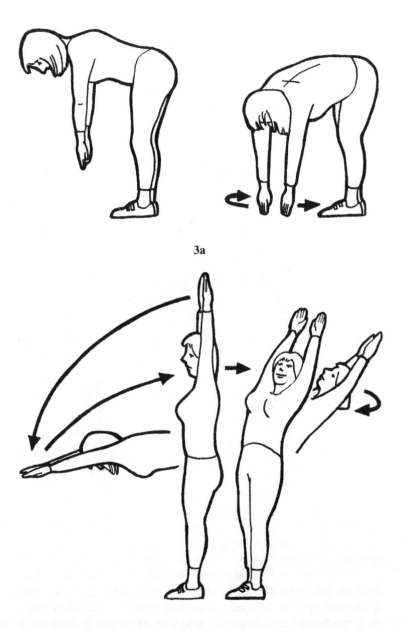

3a

3b

Exercise   4

Start in the standing position with your hands on your hips and feet parallel but slightly apart. Then bend the knees and hips, lower your heels to the floor, extending your arms for balance, and squat with your pelvis close to your heels, the shoulders being above your knees. Repeat twelve times. To make this exercise easier, hold on to a bed-rail or to a heavy article of furniture with your hands.

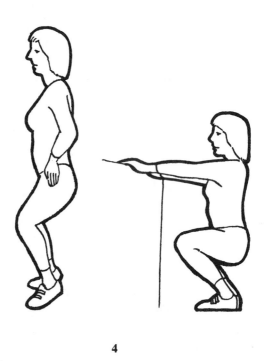

4

Exercise   5

Stand with your right hand on a bed-rail or chair-back. Kick your left leg upwards and backwards fully with a swing making an ellipse, then sideways, forwards, sideways, back and down to the starting point. Then reverse this from the back, round to the front and downwards. Repeat all movements from six to twelve times.

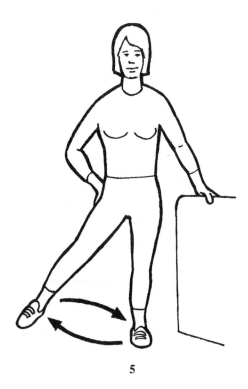

5

Exercise 6
This exercise is for the feet, and you should begin with your hands on
your hips or supported for balance:
(a) Rise and fall on your toes.
(b) Rock your ankles from side to side.
(c) Stand on your heels, raising the toes.
Repeat these exercises up to twelve times or more.

   As a variation of these foot exercises, place the ball of your foot on a
block or books three inches high, and then lower your heels to the floor.
Reverse this by placing your heels on the block and then lower your toes
to the floor. Finally, jump up and down on your toes from twelve to
twenty times.

Lying
Exercise 7
(a) Lie flat on your back with your arms at your sides. Sit up, bending

forwards towards your knees, and then return to the lying position. Repeat this three times and, as you get stronger, increase to six or more times.

(b) This exercise should be repeated with the arms extended above your head, and you should aim to reach your toes with the hands when bending forward. This modification requires extra strength and should not be forced.

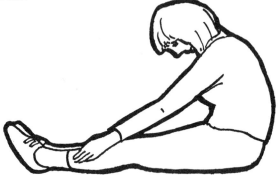

7

Exercise 8

Lie flat on your back with your legs apart and your arms extending sideways. Each hand should then reach for the opposite foot, alternately.

Exercise 9

(a) Lying on your back with your legs together, raise the legs alternately, first to a vertical position and then beyond and above the head, with knees kept straight.

(b) Then move both legs together, using your hands for support on the floor. Bring your feet to the floor beyond your head and repeat three times, increasing gradually.

Exercise 10

Lie face downwards with your hands on the floor at shoulder level, your trunk and legs straight and rigid, and your toes on the floor. Press up with your arms until they are fully extended and your body is supported on both toes and hands. Repeat this exercise three to six times, and up to twelve times as your strength increases.

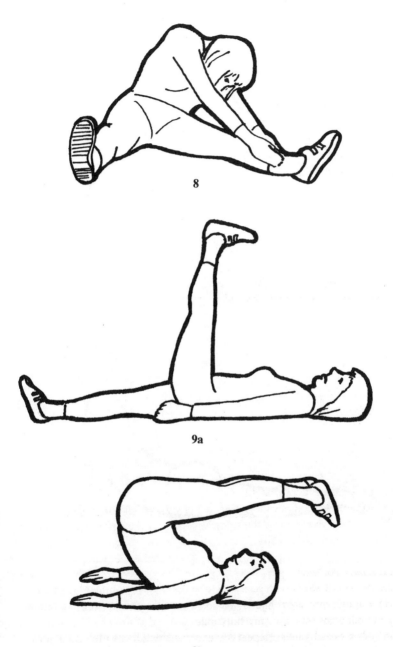

8

9a

9b

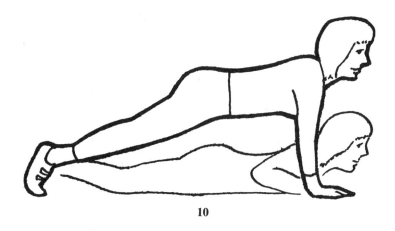

10

Exercise   11

Lie as in Exercise 10 with your legs and hips on the floor. Extend your arms till they are straight, thus raising your trunk. Repeat six times.

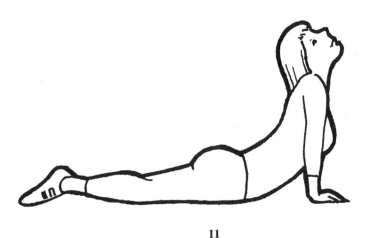

11

On hands and knees
Exercise   12

(a) Crouch on your hands and knees with your arms and knees perpendicular and your spine horizontal.

(b) Then bend your arms and lower your shoulders to the floor level, while keeping the hips high.

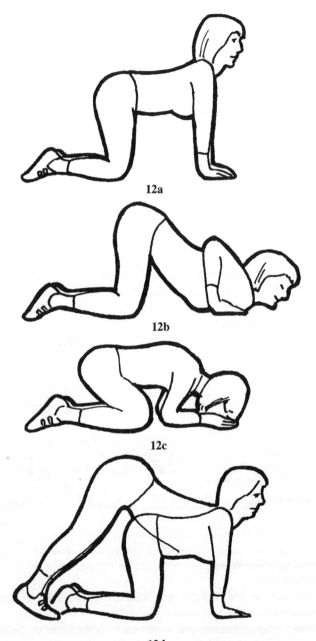

12a

12b

12c

12d

(c) Keep your shoulders low, gliding back until you are sitting on your heels. Raise your shoulders and hips once more to return to the original position (a), and repeat the exercise six to twelve times.

(d) Then recover the first position and raise and lower the lumbar spine, rocking your pelvis up and down twelve to twenty times.

Standing again
Exercise   13
(a) This exercise for pelvic rocking can be carried out either as in Exercise 12(d) or in a standing position with your feet apart and your hands on your hips as a guide to the movement. Hollow your back deeply and then straighten it, drawing the abdomen in. Then, with your legs and hands in the same position as before, and your trunk erect, rock your body from one leg to the other, repeating twelve to twenty times.

(b) To combine the above movements, stand as before, but with your knees slighly bent, and after relaxing the pelvic area, rotate the pelvis in the 'hula-hula' manner. Repeat this exercise twenty times.

The above exercises were designed to keep the body supple, but in an age when people spend most of their time sitting in offices or cars, or standing at the bench in a factory, a more vigorous approach may be required. Such a system was devised by Dr Kenneth H. Cooper and was termed by him 'aerobics'.[4]

Aerobics

Aerobics includes, among other exercises, running, swimming, cycling and jogging, and constitutes a programme to help to prevent the 'national disaster' of heart disease from which 'every year, nearly a million Americans (and many other nationals) die', and which now affects younger people and women more than it did in the past. It has been claimed that this programme lessens the chance of prematurely developing coronary heart disease or related vascular ailments and that it makes people physically and mentally alert.

The training claims to have the following effects:

'1 It strengthens the muscles of respiration and tends to reduce resistance to air flow, ultimately facilitating the rapid flow of air in and out of the lungs.

'2 It improves the strength and efficiency of the heart, enabling more blood to be pumped with each stroke. This improves the ability to more rapidly transport life-sustaining oxygen from the lungs to the heart and ultimately to all parts of the body.

'3   It tones up muscles throughout the body, thereby improving the general circulation, at times lowering blood pressure and reducing the work of the heart.
'4   It causes an increase in the total amount of blood circulating through the body and increases the number of red cells and the amount of haemoglobin, making the blood a more efficient oxygen carrier.'

Exercise charts are available for different age. groups, but an initial physical examination, especially of the heart, is essential, in order to make sure that a person is fit for the training. People are urged to stay within their tolerance when exercising and to warm up at the beginning and cool down at the end. Regularity is essential in order to build up physical fitness, and Dr Cooper's book provides useful instructions regarding the distance to run, swim or cycle, or the length of time to be spent in stationary running during the sixteen weeks when maximum efficiency is gained. There are also suggestions regarding the time to be spent playing handball, basketball and squash.[5]

Physical exercise not only helps to prevent heart disease. It also prevents further attacks after disease has struck. Findings are that 'active men appear to have two or three times less risk of myocardial infarction and two or three times greater chance of surviving a first heart attack' than inactive men.[6]

Since energy is used up during physical exercise, exercise leads to loss of weight and should be included in slimming programmes.

Another condition which calls for exercise is diabêtes, which is far more prevalent in people who lead sedentary lives than in those who are physically active. It has been found that 'the prevalence of diabetes is very low (0.1 per cent or less) in unmechanized primitive societies, rising to high levels (up to seven per cent in some cases) in under-exercising industrial communities with extended life span'.[7] Exercise is recommended for established diabetics,[8] and it has been pointed out that better circulation in the muscles during exercise leads to a decrease in blood sugar, thus tending to normalize the metabolic error which constitutes diabetes (although insulin may also be necessary in severe cases).

Autogenic training

Civilized man not only urgently needs bodily activity, but also, definitely, requires relaxation. When you hold yourself correctly in standing, sitting and walking, your posture strikes the right balance between tension and limpness - avoiding, as shown earlier, the two extremes of slumping and of a cramped position. But you must also be trained to relax completely, which is best achieved while lying down in a quiet room in semi-darkness. As is the case with exercises, there are numerous schools of thought. A successful method, which incorporates some of the yoga principles adapted for western man, was devised by J.H. Schultz. It has proved its success for many years, especially in Germany, and is known as 'Autogenic Training'. It 'improves self-regulatory functions and thus not only enhances a person's overall capacity for psychophysiological adaption but also increases bodily resistance to all kinds of stress'.[9]

If you should undergo this training, changes will be brought about in your body and mind which will affect your muscle-tone, your peripheral blood circulation, your heart-beat, your breathing and the circulation in your abdomen. You will be taught to become aware of the conditions in these parts of your body and throughout your training, auto-suggestion, aimed at achieving calmness, will be practised. Thus, as in natural therapy, vital functions on which health depends are improved, and the patient takes an active part in the training and is not treated merely as an object of medical science.

In order to reduce outside disturbances, autogenic training is carried out in a quiet, dimly-lit room, with the patient lying down or sitting in a comfortable position. You shut your eyes and are then told to suggest to yourself 'I am calm'. To achieve calmness, you have to learn to bring about the right mood, which must be maintained throughout the subsequent phases of the training. You then start the exercises concerned with the various bodily functions.

As a trainee, you first learn to achieve the sensation of heaviness, which starts in the right arm if you are right-handed, and in the left arm if you are left-handed. Gradually, calmness and heaviness merge into one experience and muscular tension is eliminated. After two to five minutes, you return to your wakeful state through a quick flexion of your elbows; this is followed by taking a deep breath and opening your eyes. Many people feel refreshed after they have been taught to relax their muscles with a feeling of calmness. After you have mastered the sensation of heaviness, you will be introduced to the next phase in which calmness and heaviness are followed by a feeling of warmth, again starting from the right or left arm. The physiological effect is on the blood vessels which become relaxed (they have their own musculature which provides the tonus of the vessel). With the sensation of warmth goes a deepening of the calming effect; feelings of heaviness and warmth fuse into one experience.

From calmness, heaviness and warmth, you proceed to influencing your heart-beat by suggesting to yourself 'my heart is beating calmly'. This experience is particularly valuable for anxious people who suffer from palpitations and from a feeling of oppression.

After having reached awareness of tranquillity through heaviness, warmth and a calm heart-beat, your attention will be concentrated on your breathing: in particular on a gentle up-and-down movement of your chest and abdomen, the movements being associated in your mind with the rhythm of life itself. (Apart from the general relaxing effect, beneficial for people in general, asthmatics in particular can expect benefit from this stage.)

When all these exercises have been perfected, the therapist will direct your attention to the stomach region and will suggest to you that the nerves around your stomach produce a feeling of warmth. Again, a variety of subjective experiences will coincide with the relaxation of your stomach; the abdominal cavity will feel alive and integrated within the calm flow of life that pervades the rest of your body.

During the last stage of this physiological - psychological training, your concentration will be focused on the forehead. Here, in contrast to the feeling of warmth which has enveloped the rest of your body, you are taught to suggest to yourself 'My forehead is slightly cool'. This pleasant sensation will add to the total experience of relaxation.

It takes from three to four months for a patient to achieve proficiency in the various stages. But with the aid of this training, you can come to terms with the tension of life and can recover from the effects of strain. Many people find that their memory and other mental functions, especially concentration, improve, as does the quality of sleep. (When the various exercises are carried out before going to sleep, the quick flexion of the elbows, the deep breathing and the opening of the eyes should be omitted.)

After you have learned to carry out the various stages of this psychosomatic training, you can be introduced to the 'high stage', which is meditative: you are told to imagine that your eyeballs are turning upwards and inwards and you are asked to imagine a colour which expresses to you a sense of harmony. You have now reached a state of contemplation and you are sinking into yourself. You become sure of your identity and you experience clarity about the meaning of your existence.

Many patients will not achieve the spiritual relaxation of this 'high stage'; some will only become adept at one of the earlier stages; for instance becoming aware of the heaviness and warmth of the body. But whatever stage is reached, autogenic training offers an antidote to the rush and tension of life.

Chapter 10

Allies to natural therapy

Homoeopathy, acupuncture, osteopathy and chiropractic are four auxiliary and independent schools of healing which share with natural therapy the common principle of trust in the whole-making integrative power of life. Also, like natural therapy, they avoid that gross interference with bodily and mental mechanisms which characterizes conventional medical science, and which can be responsible for many dangerous side-effects, while leaving uncorrected the unhealthy conditions that are largely responsible for human illness. These allies to natural therapy will now be discussed; finally, an account will be given of the relaxing and stimulating effects of massage which is another valuable addition to natural therapy.

Homoeopathy

Whereas in conventional medicine a drug is chosen for the treatment of a specific disease such as pneumonia or heart failure, the homoeopathic remedy is aimed at the *whole* person, an attitude which is in tune with natural treatment by diet, hydrotherapy, breathing exercises, and so on. The artificial division of body and mind, adopted by scientific medicine, is avoided by the homoeopathic school, and a total approach is achieved in the following way. Remedies are first given, in appropriate amounts, to healthy people. The homoeopathic doctor notes the effects of the medicines: psychological changes such as irritability and depression, and physical changes such as palpitations, contractions of the stomach, dilatation of blood vessels, etc. These objective signs are, however, not the most important features, for what interests the homoeopathic prescriber is the subjective aspect: how the person who has taken the medicine, the 'prover', experiences the changes. Is the pain in the head relieved by heat or cold, does the patient generally prefer to be warm or cool, does he feel better in the spring or in the winter, what sort of food does he like or dislike? All these and many other personal responses enter into the account which characterizes a particular remedy, the 'drug picture'.

Now, when the prescriber meets a sick person, he will enquire into the finest details of his physico-mental make-up, and will choose a remedy which will match the patient's total condition with the corresponding drug picture. Thus the *whole* patient is related to the healthy 'prover'. Like is cured by like; hence the word homoeopathy: 'homoeo' (like), 'pathy' (suffering).

The amount of drug substances in homoeopathic remedies is, as a rule, very small (thus excluding the danger of toxic effects), and the medicines are specially prepared to ensure homogeneous distribution of the material. In acute diseases, doses are given frequently - every half hour in very critical conditions, and every two to four hours in less dangerous circumstances. When the organism has responded, the homoeopathic medicine is withdrawn and, in a chronic disease, after the response has begun, no more drug stimulus is applied until the amelioration is complete.

Homoeopathic remedies are derived from the mineral, vegetable and animal kingdom. Let us look at an example of each.

A mineral substance is *natrum muriaticum,* common salt, prepared according to the rule of homoeopathy. This is used for people who have lost weight, who are irritable and reject sympathy, and who tend to suffer from throbbing headaches (in women especially during and after the period). The *natrum muriaticum* patient is constipated, the skin is often inflamed, and the patient feels better in the open air, but not in sea air.

An example of a vegetable remedy is a preparation of *anemone-pulsatilla.* In contrast to the previous picture, here we have a patient who is weepy and craves for sympathy, whose symptoms change frequently, and whose pains shift from one place to another. The patient suffers from digestive upsets after eating rich food and, although the mouth is dry, is not thirsty. In women, the periods are scanty and irregular. Sleep is delayed and restless, a warm room or a close atmosphere is not tolerated, and fresh air is a necessity.

Snake venom, *lachesis,* is one of the remedies derived from the animal kingdom, and is given especially to women who are suspicious, have a vivid imagination and are loquacious. The troubles which occur at the change of life, the irritability and the flushes, are often helped by this remedy. *Lachesis* patients feel worse before the period (which may be irregular during the change), but better when the flow is established. There is a tendency to bleed from small wounds. This drug cures conditions which are similar to those induced by a snake bite.

The number of drugs available is constantly being increased. Some drug pictures are far more complete than others. The material medica comprises several thousands of remedies. But homoeopathy also has its limitations. The therapist has to keep other measures in readiness if the patient requires them; an urgent operation may have to be performed in the case of a perforated stomach ulcer, a deficiency may have to be made good as is the case in diabetes when insulin must be given, or a weakened heart may need digitalis, and so on. Apart from such urgent needs for scientific medicine, the limitations of homoeopathy lie in its dependence on the possibility of matching the patient's personality with a detailed drug picture. The greater the similarity of the patient's condition to one of the known drug pictures, the better are the chances of helping him.

How does the homoeopathic remedy act? Not through the drug substance as a conventional pharmacological agent. According to the homoeopathic school, the remedy acts through the healing power of nature, evident in the patient's response. This, of course, accords with the basic tenet of natural therapy. Thus the two schools are complementary.[1] Dr Samuel Hahnemann, the founder of homoeopathic medicine, accepted natural therapy; he insisted that a patient's mode of living, including his diet, must be corrected before the stimulus of the homoeopathic medicine can be expected to effect a cure.

Having discovered the appropriate homoeopathic medicine, it can be of assistance in the choice of the correct natural stimulus. For instance, responses to heat and cold form essential features in homoeopathic drug pictures. It follows that a patient whose medicine has been worked out to be a remedy suitable for chilly people cannot be expected to respond to cold-water treatment. The three examples, given above, *natrum muriaticum, anemone,* and *lachesis* are all remedies which fit people who can stand cold temperatures well, but a *natrum muriaticum* patient cannot tolerate sea air, hence the natural therapist may advocate as a change of scenery a stay in the country or in the mountains.

In the homoeopathic drug picture we may find a combination of afflictions of the skin, such as eczema, and in the chest, such as asthma. The remedy, amorphous carbon, will tend to be helpful for both conditions, thus restoring the disturbed equilibrium which the natural therapist restores by his use of natural stimuli.

Temporary aggravations are expected by both the natural therapy and the homoeopathic schools. The possible beneficial 'cleaning' effect of an attack of diarrhoea was mentioned earlier (page 33), and under homoeopathic treatment such healing responses are often brought about soon after a remedy has been given. Such a reaction confirms that the drug was chosen correctly.

Homoeopathic and conventional medicine meet in the prevention of specific infections, although they differ on dosage and methods of application. The conventional school carries out immunization against such infectious illnesses as diphtheria, whooping cough and influenza, and particular toxins are injected into the patient in order to stimulate the formation of antibodies and to prevent an attack of the disease. The homoeopathic school uses dilutions of the poison of these infections in order either to prevent an attack or to help the patient to recover from the after-effects of one.

As regards the difference in dosage, the small or infinitesimal dose is not an essential feature of homoeopathic medicine; homoeopathy's fundamental tenet is the matching of the remedy with the patient. It is, however, true that many homoeopathic physicians prescibe 'potencies' which lie outside the molecular limit; this means that, for instance, a 30. potency of sulphur does not contain any sulphur. The homoeopath, however, claims that it contains some energy derived from the original sulphur which has now entered the medium in which the sulphur was diluted (for instance, spirit or sugar), and which could manifest itself through specific sulphur radiations.

All this is speculation. The homoeopath points out that the efficacy of his preparations, including the high potencies, has been proved empirically over more than 150 years. And, although some of these 'potencies' do not contain any of the material from which they were derived, it does not follow that they are ineffective. Let us remember that modern physicists do not hold that, ultimately, the universe consists of matter. From a philosophical point of view, it must be pointed out that matter, molecules and energy of concepts created by the scientist's mind and are not part of the reality of nature. The world, apart from the knowing mind, is inscrutable.[2]

Acupuncture

By dropping a few granules of sugar, impregnated with a specially diluted remedy on a patient's tongue, the homoeopath sets nature's vitalizing power into motion. Similarly, by touching certain points on a patient's skin with a fine needle, the acupuncturist mobilizes the same force.

Acupuncture has been practised in China for thousands of years, and the Chinese explain its efficacy in a metaphysical way. They maintain that the unity of life embodies a negative principle, Yin, and a positive principle Yang. An assumption of the existence of these two forces is not confined to the field of biology, but pervades the whole of Chinese life and is found in art, literature and philosophy. The interplay of Yin and Yang is traced as a rhythmical movement throughout the universe, which is explained in this polar manner; any disturbance of the relationship between the two poles constitutes disharmony, which in medicine stands for disease.

The acupuncturist defines channels through which the life energy flows: they are the 'meridians' which follow a well-defined course on the body surface. By inserting fine needles into these 'meridians' he claims that the disturbed balance can be restored and a cure brought about. The natural therapist steeped in western thought, cannot accept the dualistic metaphysical conception but he can accept the concept of harmony standing for health and wholeness. He might explain the effects of the pricking of the skin in terms of a reflex. The skin is richly supplied with nerves, and these are connected with the spinal cord, with the brain, and, indirectly, with all the organs in the body.[3] For instance, tension of the muscles in the back, distorting the spine and thus affecting the rest of the body, can be relieved by acupuncture. In this way, great help can be given to the vast number of people who suffer from backache. Such patients are not only physically tense, they also suffer from emotional tension, and by the use of acupuncture both forms of tension may be removed.[4]

The acupuncturist accepts relationships between the skin and the internal organs in a way which differs from the teachings of the medical schools. For instance, he considers that a disturbed liver causes migraine, allergic conditions, gout, poor eyesight and general tiredness and weakness. He asserts that by stimulating the liver through the skin, all these conditions can be cured. From the point of view of natural therapy, the liver is of importance as the large detoxicating organ; thus, acupuncture, directed to the liver meridian, may assist the cleansing efforts which are encouraged during a fast or an eliminative diet. Since the days of the ancient Greeks, the liver, the producer of the gall, has been associated with a 'choleric' temperament. A natural therapist is aware of the emotional effects of a toxic physical condition. Similarly, the Chinese acupuncturist refers to the liver as 'the seat of the Unconscious'; thus, by treating the liver, he is convinced that he treats the mind.[5]

Some modern western medical acupuncturists also claim to influence the mind directly. Dr Paul Renard, for instance, has related acupuncture to the tenets of the various schools of psychological medicine, and, at the same time, to the drug pictures of certain homoeopathic remedies.[6] We have seen that homoeopathy also considers the patient as a psychosomatic unit, and the relationship between acupuncture and homoeopathy is accepted by other French acupuncturists besides Renard.

Following Renard, we may assume that the mind is 'accessible' to the acupuncturist, as he has proved that he can deeply influence the nervous system, that he can abolish the sensation of pain to such a degree that major operations can be carried out without any ordinary anaesthetic. A modification of brain activity may well amount to a change in mental activity.

The Chinese acupuncturist pays great attention to the pulse and is trained to feel fourteen different pulses above the wrist. In this way, he judges the conditions of the organs throughout the body.

Dr Otto Bergsmann, working with Dr J. Bischko at the Vienna Institute for the Study of Acupuncture (das Ludwig-Boltzmann Institut für Akupunktur), has related certain points situated on the skin to certain pathological processes in the lungs. These authors have explained the effect of acupuncture in terms of a *regulation* of bodily activities, and they have developed new methods which are suitable for this type of research.[7] This is an example of integrating the knowledge gained by Chinese workers into the field of scientific medicine. As we have seen, a regulative force is postulated also by homoeopathy and by natural therapy; it is a manifestation of nature's vital force. It is also a fundamental concept in the systems of osteopathy and chiropractic, further allies of natural therapy.

Osteopathy

The manipulations which are used in conjunction with the methods of natural therapy belong to the special field of *osteopathy* and *chiropractic*. The principles of osteopathy have been interpreted within the conceptual framework of modern sciences,[8] and the effects of this mechanical treatment can be understood in terms of cybernetics, the science which is concerned with controls and communications within a system. It is thought that equilibrium is achieved by 'negative feedback': part of the output of surplus energy is diverted in order to achieve a balance. In the living organism, communications between different parts occur through reflex activity, and disturbances in this channel can be the result of mechanical faults such as sprains, obstructions of lymph and blood vessels, and immobilization of joints. Any disturbance in the bodily structure which is apt to lead to a disturbance of function is called an osteopathic lesion or a facilitated segment and since it affects muscles and bones, is is 'musculoskeletal'. The disturbance may consist of a restriction of mobility within a section of the spine, interfering with the reflexes that extend from the spinal column to other parts of the body, including the internal organs. The lesion interrupts the feedback and a correction by the osteopath restores normal functioning of the dynamic pattern. Not only does the mechanical fault cause biochemical disturbances in the tissues, a biochemical disturbance can itself cause mechanical malfunctioning. Such biochemical faults may result from a disturbed function of a nerve and may be amenable to manipulations of the spine. Thus, the osteopath claims that he can release spasm in the intestines, regulate the heart-beat and correct abnormal circulation in different parts of the body.

Two types of osteopathic lesion are distinguished: the primary lesion resulting from an abnormal stimulus originating in the spine which has caused some alteration within the body, and the secondary osteopathic lesion which has developed as the outcome of some visceral irritation or other abnormal functioning within the organism. The result is a faulty posture which causes pain and tenderness in the affected areas. The body responds to the irritation with alteration in elasticity, in fluid content, in texture, in temperature, in colour, in vascular supply and in abnormal electrical conditions. Experiments on animals are said to have confirmed the theory of the osteopathic lesion and its physiological consequences, and further evidence has been collected through examining the changes in the muscles and nerves of human beings.

The osteopath uses technical manoeuvres which affect the various parts of the body: lymphatic drainage through special massage, movements of the chest wall which affect the heart and the blood vessels inside the chest, and manipulation of joints with special reference to the vertebral column. It is also claimed that manipulative therapy 'can play a major role' in the treatment of ulcers in the stomach and duodenum. In case of inflammation in the kidneys, the correction of osteopathic lesions is said to improve the circulation and thus assist in the healing. Manipulative osteopathic treatment to the lower part of the spine is employed for the relief of bladder troubles,and allergic diseases are said to respond to manipulations of the spine, as such manipulations reduce the exaggerated sensitivity which is the cause of the condition. Bronchial asthma is one of the allergic conditions for which an osteopathic technique has been devised.[9]

While employing specific techniques, osteopathic treatment relies on the integration of the whole body; in this respect osteopaths accept the fundamental conception of natural therapy. They also admit limitations to their system of healing, and accept the need for the conventional methods of scientific medicine in some conditions.

Chiropractic

The word chiropractic is derived from two Greek words, 'cheir' (hand) and 'practikos' which means manual practice. Chiropractors employ a wide range of manual techniques to treat spinal and other joints. Treatment is mainly for pain in the back, the neck, the head and in various joints. Like all natural medicines, chiropractic emphasizes the body's own healing mechanisms. Chiropractors are chiefly concerned with spinal joint dysfunction and with its frequent effect on the proper functioning of the nervous system which is intimately linked to the spine.

Chiropractic, though not well known in Britain, is recognized in many countries, with nearly 50,000 practitioners worldwide.[10]

Massage

Massage can either be given to the patient by a professional person or the patient can be taught to massage himself.

Professional massage

Spinal manipulations are often combined with massage which is chiefly applied to the large muscles situated on either side of the spine. The beneficial effects of acupuncture are also improved if the muscular relaxation which is achieved by the insertion of the fine needles is followed by firm rubbing.

Acupuncture effects can, in fact, be achieved by massage of the points into which the acupuncturist inserts his needles, these areas being 'trigger points', sensitive areas from which nervous impulses travel to other parts of the body. Thus massage not only relieves local conditions such as sprains, congestion and tension, but also influences parts of the body which are connected by reflexes with the area which is massaged. A general massage provides relaxation and is of physical and psychological benefit. Mrs Elisabeth Dicke has discovered a further important use. Her technique consists in pushing the skin with the third and fourth fingers against underlying tissues such as bone, tendons and muscles. The resulting pull constitutes a stimulus which affects the nervous system, the blood and lymph, and the cells situated under the skin which are concerned with drainage of waste products deposited in the tissues. Dicke found that areas which had become hardened could become soft again, and that remarkable relief could be given to patients suffering from a disturbance of circulation. Her connective tissue massage always starts at the base of the spine and extends upwards. [11]

Self-massage

Apart from receiving treatment from a trained person, people can apply massage to their own bodies. They can discover areas of *muscular tension,* especially below the collar bones, over the buttocks and on the upper inner parts of their thighs. Through firm, deep massage the tension can be relieved. The massage is painful at first, but as the hardness is overcome the pain goes and the relief is felt on distant parts of the body. One area which is not accessible to the fingers but which is often the seat of tension is the shoulder blades. This part can be massaged by leaning and rubbing against the raised edges of a door. Musicians, who frequently strain the muscles of their forearms and consequently have to stop playing because of pain, can get rid of their tensions by massage, applied to tense muscles in various parts of their bodies, and can resume playing.

Massage techniques for the abdomen, the legs, and the tonsillar region will now be described and, finally, it will be suggested how the whole body can benefit from vigorous brushing or towelling.

Self-massage of abdomen

This form of massage aims at stimulating the bowels and is therefore helpful in constipation and flatulence. (It should not be used in cases of inflammation, which are often characterized by pain.) The patient lies on the back with the knees flexed. The right hand presses against the right lower part of the abdomen while the left hand, lying on top of the right hand, increases the pressure. Now, both hands move upwards towards the ribs, then across the stomach to the left side, and then downwards. This whole movement is performed while breathing out. The breath is taken in while the hands resume their starting position on the right side. The movements are repeated fifteen to twenty times.

Another type of abdominal self-massage consists in using the fingers of the right hand as a hammer which, through movements of the wrist, taps against the various parts of the abdomen. The tapping should be very gentle in the upper part where the stomach is situated and should not be applied to the part in the centre, where the bladder lies. The tapping takes place while breathing out, and follows the same route as the abdominal massage described earlier.

Abdominal self-massage can be carried out very effectively without using the hands, by a jerking movement of the abdominal muscles. The position is the same as when self-massage of the abdomen is given. The abdomen is drawn in and jerked out. This in-and-out movement is repeated fifteen to twenty times. The back does not move and is not raised. The breathing rhythm is not disturbed; inspiration takes place during two to four of the flicker movements, expiration during four to six. It is important that the quick movements of the diaphragm do not interfere with proper breathing. If carried out correctly, this form of self-massage is very beneficial for those conditions which respond to ordinary abdominal self-massage. (The same precautions obtain with regard to inflammatory diseases.)

Self-massage of legs

The person lies on the back and bends the right leg so that the right foot can be grasped with both hands. Both hands then begin the self-massage from the toes, with stroking movements which extend upwards beyond the knee. These movements are repeated about five times and then the calf is shaken vigorously with both hands, starting from the heel and going up to the knee. The calf muscles are further relaxed through hacking movements, using the edge of the fifth finger and the adjacent part of the hand, again starting from the heel. Now the muscles of the thigh are firmly stroked with both hands in an upward direction, and then shaken. Next, hacking movements are applied to the thigh in the same manner as to the calf. Several large stroking movements from the toes to the hips complete the massage, which is then repeated on the left leg. The self-massage aids the circulation in the legs and is also used in cases of cramps. It should not be used where there is inflammation, or in cases of varicose veins since clots situated in the veins could be dislodged and cause serious disturbances in other parts of the circulatory system.

Self-massage of tonsils

The tonsils and the surrounding tissues belong to the lymphatic system; this is concerned with the mobilization of defences against invading micro-organisms. Natural therapists assume that the tonsils are related to various glands within the body, to the organs concerned with digestion of food, and to the nervous system - especially to certain parts of the brain. Thus, tonsillar massage has far-reaching stimulating effects. It also aids the clearing of material which has accumulated in the tonsillar crypts, and it can be helpful in cases of catarrh in the upper part of the throat. The massage is carried out with the index finger. If the tonsils are inflamed, the treatment should not be applied, as it could lead to an aggravation of the inflammation which might affect other parts of the body, especially the kidneys. Tonsillar massage can be made more effective by means of suction applied through a glass tube and operated by means of a rubber bulb.

Whole-body brushing or rough towelling

Vigorous brushing or rough towelling can stimulate the skin and, indirectly, the whole body. The treatment starts from the right arm and is directed towards the heart. Next, the left arm is treated, followed by the front of the body, and then the back. Finally, the feet and legs are rubbed.

Chapter 11

Twelve case histories

Natural therapy and its auxiliary methods will now be illustrated by quoting twelve cases. Although each has been identified with the name of an illness, it should be remembered that treatment, which is based on the idea of wholeness, is not so much given for the specific disease as for the patient who suffers from it. In each case, the question asked was: in what respect has the patient, in his or her mode of living, neglected the principles on which health (i.e. wholeness) depends? In trying to restore the patient to health (wholeness), the therapist had to assess what response to the natural methods could be expected.

Case 1: Recurrent boils

A man of 42 had been plagued with boils for seven years. They had started near his left ear but had then affected the sweat glands in his armpits. He had received enormous amounts of penicillin, also X-ray treatment, and an incision had been made in his left axilla. Finally, a major operation by a plastic surgeon - the removal of a large part of the affected skin - had been advised.

The natural therapist enquired into the patient's diet - something which had never been done before. It transpired that this man was in the habit of taking ten cups of tea per day, putting four teaspoonsful of sugar into each. In addition, he drank coffee sweetened with sugar, enjoyed carbohydrates such as jam, puddings and sweet biscuits, and smoked 40 to 60 cigarettes a day.

The treatment consisted in the elimination of all sugar, coffee and tea, and the man was told that he must stop smoking. He was put on a diet: mostly raw fruit and vegetables with cottage cheese and yoghurt as protein. He also received a homoeopathic medicine, *Hepar Sulphuris,* which is helpful in cases of boils.

The patient made excellent progress. In the first two weeks his weight dropped from 12 stone 2 lb (77.2 kg) to 11 stone 10lb (74.5 kg). He felt better in himself and the inflammation in his armpits was much reduced. He still craved for cigarettes, however, and smoked about three per day. The man's diet was now increased by three eggs a week, two Ryvita biscuits per day, and ordinary cheese.

Four weeks after the start of the treatment, his weight had become steady, and the boils were small (whereas before there had been large collections of pus). In order to increase his protein intake, nuts were added to the diet. The patient was by now convinced that the new regime was beneficial, and his full co-operation was won. Eight months after the start of the treatment he was allowed meat, fish and cooked vegetables in addition to his original diet. The inflammation in his armpits decreased, so that after one year no more boils appeared. Four and a half years after his first consultation with the natural therapist, his local doctor reported that there had not been any recurrence of boils.

The natural therapist treated this patient's disease by eliminating harmful habits and recommending a diet which consisted largely of uncooked vegetables and fruit. Dairy produce was introduced from the beginning and later, meat and fish. Thus the body recovered its powers to deal with the germs which are present on every skin but which, in this case, had caused serious trouble.

Case 2: Ulcerative colitis and recurrent virus infection of the skin

A man had suffered in his childhood from frequent attacks of influenza, bronchitis, and from a prolonged fever which had presumably been caused by a virus. At the age of 19, he started having attacks of diarrhoea. At the age of 23, there was blood in his stools and the diagnosis of ulcerative colitis was made. With the diarrhoea he had bouts of fever which weakened him considerably and he also suffered abdominal pain. At the age of 28, he had his first attack of herpes simplex, a virus infection of the skin, which recurred frequently and was each time accompanied by looseness of his bowels, loss of appetite and general malaise.

Homoeopathic treatment started when he was 29, and the remedy, *pyrogen,* which is prepared from septic material, precipitated an attack of diarrhoea accompanied by fever, but then led to recovery from his bowel trouble. Other homoeopathic medicines, such as *cinchona* (Peruvian bark), were also helpful, but his herpes simplex continued to trouble him, causing considerable weakness. At the age of 33, he consulted a natural therapist, and in view of his long history, his determination to achieve better health, and his youth, a strict dietetic regime was suggested:

Breakfast
2 grated apples + 2 tablespoonsful of oats soaked in 4 tablespoonsful of water overnight + 1 carton of yoghurt + 1 dessertspoonful of Froment. Apple juice, herb tea.

Lunch
Raw salad without salt and vinegar, oil, lemon juice, Ryvita biscuit, vegetarian margarine, cottage cheese.

Tea-time
Apple juice.

Supper
Another raw salad with fruit, potato in jacket, yoghurt.

Water treatment was also prescribed: a cold sponge of the whole body, morning and night. Later he increased his vitality by carrying out Dr Kenneth Cooper's 'aerobics'. He also received further homoeopathic medicines from time to time.

The patient felt the impact of this frugal way of living and was frightened by the response from his friends who warned him that he would lose strength. When visiting them, he felt that, by rejecting their food, he had rejected them. But, gradually, the patient and his friends got used to the situation, and he so much liked the food that he had no wish to return to his former diet. After three weeks, cooked vegetables were added in the form of 'Vecon', a vegetable powder, to be dissolved in hot water. The soup was thickened and made more nourishing by the addition of unpolished rice.

Under natural therapy, the patient experienced immediate relief from an irritation of the skin which had worried him considerably and which had seriously interfered with his sleep. This symptom was interpreted as an expression of his toxic state. The first ten days were difficult; for his body had not learnt to assimilate the food and he felt rather hungry. Then a reaction set in: he suffered from headache, felt very weak, perspired heavily, felt thirsty but not hungry. This was a crisis which was a turning point in his illness. After that, his general condition improved, his sense of taste and of smell improved considerably, he felt less tense, calmer and more energetic, and was looking forward to his work. His bowels recovered except for a short bout of diarrhoea. His attacks of herpes became much milder, and no longer depressed and exhausted him. Natural therapy had raised his resistance.

This man's case is instructive because, although he had made progress after homoeopathic treatment, he gained a greater measure of health after adopting a natural therapy regime.

Case 3: Osteo-arthritis

A woman of sixty-one, weighing 12 stone 6 lb (79 kg) complained that during the past fifteen months she had suffered from pain in her knees which the doctor had diagnosed as osteo-arthritis. She had been ordered tablets for the pain, but they had not given her much relief.

An inquiry into her diet revealed that she ate wholemeal bread, marmalade, Ryvita, cheese, eggs, fruit, meat, fish and yoghurt, and that she drank tea and decaffeinated coffee. She was asked to give up bread, was put on a lacto-vegetarian diet, and was encouraged to sponge her whole body with cold water, morning and night. After three weeks, she had lost seven pounds (3 kg) and her knee was more comfortable. The knee improved further, she lost another five pounds (2.25 kg) and was able to walk with comfort four and a half months after she had started treatment.

This patient was told that she had to be careful not to gain weight. The treatment was not drastic, but the change in her mode of living proved sufficient to bring about marked improvement.

Case 4: Varicose ulcers

A woman aged 49 and weighing 13 stone 7 lb (85.8 kg), complained of ulcers on her legs. They had first appeared when she was only 12 years old. They had scarred over and for the next 25 years remained healed. When she was 37, she developed an ulcer on her left leg. She attended a natural therapist, who prescribed a lacto-vegetarian diet, on which she lost five pounds (2.25 kg). The leg was bandaged to support the venous circulation, homoeopathic medicines were prescribed, and the ulcer gradually diminished in size, healing after one year and nine months.

Eight years later two large ulcers appeared, exuding foul pus. It was decided to admit her to hospital, and to put her on a fast. Tests were carried out to make sure that her heart was fit and that there were no deficiencies in her blood. For twelve days she had only water to drink and was given some vitamins; during this period she lost 21 pounds (9.5 kg) and the ulcers healed. The case was followed up. Two years after the fast, she reported that every second week she had fasted every other day for 24 hours and had thus succeeded in keeping her weight down to a level two stone (12.7 kg) less than it had been before the fast. There was no recurrence of ulceration and she was fit.

Case 5: Cirrhosis of the liver

A middle-aged woman developed jaundice, was admitted to hospital, and diagnosis of cirrhosis of the liver was made. She stayed in hospital for nine weeks and was given cortisone for the following two years. As this drug upset her severely, she refused to take any more. The next year, she put herself on a grape diet for four weeks, eating only several pounds of grapes per day. While on grapes, she felt well and lost the discomfort in her abdomen which had disturbed her before. Her discomfort recurred, however, when she went back to ordinary food.

Two years later she repeated the grape cure on her own, eating four to five pounds (approximately 2 kg) of grapes per day for another four weeks. Again her discomfort disappeared and she felt well, while she lost 21 lbs (9.5 kg) in weight. She then went back to a conventional diet.

As she felt ill again, she consulted a natural therapist. She was given a diet which consisted of Weetabix, milk, and orange juice for breakfast; vegetable soup, wholemeal bread and cheese for lunch; and a salad with cheese, occasional eggs, baked potato and some milk for supper. In addition, she received a homoeopathic medicine, made from the Water Ash. (This remedy is suitable for patients with liver and digestive upsets, and thus suited the patient's condition.) Under this dietetic and homoeopathic treatment, the patient made rapid progress, lost her discomfort, and gained four pounds (1.8 kg) in one month.

Conventional medicine has no special treatment for cirrhosis of the liver and patients are not given a special diet although they are advised to avoid alcohol. In this case, a small piece of liver tissue (biopsy) had been examined and the diagnosis had been confirmed. The patient had been told that her condition was likely to improve, but this did not occur until natural therapy, which included the use of the appropriate homoeopathic remedy, was instituted.

Case 6: A catarrhal child

A little girl, aged two, was brought to a natural therapist with a history of frequent colds, constant thick yellow nasal discharge, and frequent attacks of ear-ache. She was put on a diet consisting of muesli, lemon juice and honey for breakfast; cheese salad and fruit for lunch; and meat or fish, cooked vegetables, potatoes in their skins, and fruit for supper. When she was seen about three years later, the mother reported that there had been no more colds nor any nasal discharge while she was on the diet, but that she had recently started eating school lunches and had also deviated from her diet when invited to other children's homes where white bread and cakes were provided. The catarrh in her nose had returned and blocked her nostrils, tending to make her breathe through her mouth.

The natural therapist gave a certificate to enable the child to take a packed salad lunch to school, and also instructed the mother to encourage the child to breathe through her nose, to remind her of it during the day, and if possible, to close her mouth with a firm elastic strap under the chin at night. In addition, she received a homoeopathic medicine, *Silica 30.*

This case illustrates a common problem. Children are subjected to operations on their tonsils and adenoids and are given antibodies for coughs and ear-ache, when the correct treatment is in fact a reform of their diet, a cutting out of white flour, eaten as pastry and white bread, and of sugar, consumed in sweets. School lunches and the conventional teas offered to children at home, especially at parties, are a potent factor in keeping the catarrhal condition going, and this case shows how difficult it is for a child to remain a member of his or her group and still to continue on a healthy diet.

Case 7: Rheumatoid arthritis

A woman aged 38 was taken ill with swellings of many joints and a fever. She was diagnosed as a case of acute rheumatoid arthritis, lost 21 lbs (9.5 kg) in weight, and became very weak and anaemic. She was discharged from a hospital where she had not made any progress, and was first seen by a natural therapist two years after the onset of the illness. He found that the joints in her arms and legs were swollen and painful. The skin on her face was inflamed, there were cracks at the corners of her mouth, scaling on her scalp and her nails were brittle. She coughed and brought up some yellow phlegm. She was constipated. She had ceased to menstruate. An inquiry into her diet showed that it had been conventional: she had bacon and eggs, bread, butter and milk for breakfast; vegetables, meat, and grilled tomatoes for lunch; sometimes fish, tomatoes, bread, butter, milk and egg for tea; and bread and milk for supper.

The natural therapist modified her diet by reducing the meat to twice a week, ordering yoghurt as the main form of protein, introducing more raw vegetables, but also allowing some cooked vegetables, and adding oats and blackcurrant puree as an additional source of vitamin C. After the first week, he reduced the meat to once a week and then cut it out completely. For further protein, she took soya preparations and nut cream, and was also allowed brown unpolished rice.

Her knees had become fixed in a flexed state. In order to straighten them, a pulley was fixed to the end of her bed and weights were attached. To help the functions of her skin, she was sponged all over with lukewarm water three times a day. She was given a homoeopathic medicine which helps patients with arthritis - a dilution of the poison oak.

Her bowels became regular, her knees straight and her fever subsided, but her skin remained inflamed and itchy. Two further homoeopathic remedies helped her in this respect - petroleum and the spurge olive. Her stools were cultured to investigate her bowel flora, and the next homoeopathic remedy consisted of a dilution of the prevalent organisms: bacillus proteus. This last prescription caused some aggravation in the pain of her joints but she soon felt better, and thus the reaction was beneficial. Her joints improved and her cough lessened.

This treatment had commenced in May of one year and by the January of the next her menstrual period returned, another sign of a general recovery. By February of that year, her knees had become straight, she could move them normally and she started to walk again. By April her chest was clear. In June her stools became loose and she reported that the pain in her joints was relieved by passing the motion. Thus, no attempt was made to control the diarrhoea, as it was obviously helping in the healing process. By April of the following year, the patient was sleeping better, she could walk for forty-five minutes, and had gained two stone (12.7 kg) in weight, and her skin was practically normal. She received several further homoeopathic medicines, amongst them a preparation made from the cuttle fish, which improved her emotional state.

The patient kept in touch with her therapist for the next thirty-nine years. Her arthritis never caused her any marked disability. She led an active life, got married and was able to look after a big house. She never deviated from her lacto-vegetarian diet.

This case demonstrates the beneficial effects of natural therapy in a patient crippled with rheumatoid arthritis. As was pointed out in the first chapter, this condition is very common and the sufferers are mostly treated with drugs to relieve their pain. In contrast to such purely symptomatic palliative treatment, natural therapy gets to the root of the trouble and restores health by stimulating the defences of the body. The patient's progress showed how the skin, the linings of the bronchial tubes and the micro-organisms in the bowels were all involved, and how their condition was improved by the natural methods. The looseness of the bowel was interpreted as a healing effort to eliminate toxic material. The patient's attitude was of vital importance. By adopting natural therapy as her new way of life, she obtained lasting benefit.

Case 8: Heart failure

A man of 67 was admitted to hospital with a heart attack (occlusion of one of the blood vessels within the heart muscle). He was discharged after three weeks, suffering from breathlessness and swollen ankles, signs of heart failure.

He then consulted a natural therapist, who found that his breakfast consisted of four cups of tea with milk and sugar, his lunch of white bread sandwiches with cheese, tomatoes and lettuce, and his supper of meat or fish with vegetables. This diet was drastically changed. For the first two weeks he was allowed only raw vegetables, Weetabix, yoghurt and cheese. He was told to sponge his whole body with cold water, and he received a homoeopathic medicine, sulphur, which suited his constitution.

There was an immediate improvement and he found he could walk without getting breathless. After one month he was allowed some cooked vegetables and an occasional egg. After two months, he reported that he could walk for two and a half miles without getting breathless or tired. His weight had dropped from 12 stone (75.5 kg) to 10 stone 2 lb (64.5 kg), and had now stabilized. Further foods - honey, Ryvita biscuits, wholemeal bread, some milk, and meat three times a week - were added two weeks later.

This case demonstrates that natural therapy can be of great benefit in cases of heart failure and that after an initial strict regime, the patient can be allowed a fairly full diet, provided white flour and sugar are excluded.

Case 9: Advanced nephritis

A young man aged 24 was taken ill with the signs of an inflammation of his kidneys (nephritis). He had albumen in his urine and evidence of kidney disease in his blood. He was treated by an eminent specialist in kidney diseases. The illness advanced to a chronic state and the patient's father was informed that chances of a cure were minimal. The only conventional treatment consisted of prolonged rest in bed and avoidance of salt in the diet, but this regime did not make any difference to the patient's condition.

He had eaten the usual type of food - meat, fish, white bread - and had drunk tea and coffee. As he was determined to try natural therapy, he put himself on a stricter diet consisting of fruit and orange juice for breakfast, brown bread sandwiches with egg, cheese and marmite for lunch, orange juice at tea-time, and meat, fish, eggs, macaroni, vegetables, pastry and fruit for supper.

He began treatment with a natural therapist two months later, when he was given a very strict diet: muesli and raw vegetables only. He was encouraged to take air and sun baths and was instructed in breathing exercises. He also received a homoeopathic medicine, *Kali Arsenicosum,* which benefits sufferers from nephritis. There was a quick response to the combined natural and homoeopathic treatments; he felt better in himself. Then his stools became loose and offensive; this was interpreted as an effort on the part of his body to eliminate toxic material, and no attempt was made to stop the diarrhoea.

After three months, there was some objective improvement; the excretion of albumen in his urine had diminished. Another homoeopathic medicine, also helpful in kidney diseases, *Kali Iodatum,* was prescribed. The looseness of the bowels persisted for some time, while the general condition improved.

After seven months on natural treatment, he was still feeling rather tense. Autogenic training was begun; the patient learned to relax and to experience heaviness, warmth, calm heart action, calm breathing, and warmth in the nerve centre of the abdomen. Eleven months after the start of the treatment, his weight had increased from 8 stone 5½ lb (53.5 kg) - at the beginning of the treatment - to 9 stone 1 lb (57.5 kg). At that time, some cream cheese and wholemeal bread were added to the diet. Eight months later he introduced cooked vegetables and yoghurt as well as eggs and nuts into his diet, and six months later there was no longer any albumen in his urine.

This patient remained on a lacto-vegetarian diet and had at least one raw salad meal every day. He had regular checkups for his kidney trouble and the last thorough examination was carried out when he was 45, 21 years from the start of his natural therapy treatment. He was assured that he was completely cured.

A case of advanced inflammation of the kidneys, for which there was no treatment in conventional scientific medicine, was cured by natural therapy including homoeopathy and autogenic training. The patient's excellent co-operation made the prolonged strict treatment possible.

Case 10: Acne vulgaris
The acne started in this girl's case at the age of 12 when her menstrual periods commenced. Ointments and exposure to artifical ultraviolet light and even to X-rays were tried. When she was 19, she attended the skin department of the Royal London Homoeopathic Hospital. By then her face was severely disfigured by redness, pustules, large bags of pus and thick scar formation. There were also pustules on her chest and back. She received homoeopathic medicines, a high dilution of the common salt (*natrum muriaticum*) and of sulphur. There was some improvement, but as she had not changed her eating habits, the improvement did not last. For the next two and a half years, she took an antibiotic which kept her condition under control. Then she had to stop the drug, as the side-effects had become too disturbing.

The turning point in this case was reached when the girl's diet was changed. She had been consuming too much carbohydrate: her breakfast had consisted of Bran Flakes and coffee, her lunch of biscuits and Energen bread, her evening meal of meat, vegetables and a sweet. The natural therapist decided that a strict regime was necessary and that the emphasis should lie on raw fruit and raw vegetables. Breakfast was altered to a mixture of oats, apples, froment and yoghurt, a modification of the muesli; lunch and the evening meal consisted of raw salad, cottage cheese and a potato in its skin or a piece of Ryvita. As it was winter, vegetable soup was allowed to keep her warm, but tea and coffee were excluded. This strict diet was kept up for six weeks, when other items were introduced, but pastry, chocolate and fried foods were eaten only seldom. Raw and cooked vegetables remained important items in her diet. A number of homoeopathic medicines were prescribed: *kali bromatum*, which has a close relationship to acne pustules; a mixture of sulphur, silica and vegetable charcoal which is beneficial in septic conditions in general, and sulphur in a high dilution which has a deep constitutional effect.

The result of this combined natural and homoeopathic treatment was highly satisfactory; the bags of pus and pustules went and the skin assumed a normal texture. There was also a marked improvement in the patient's general health: she lost previous pains in her head and back and also an unpleasant taste, a sign of elimination of toxins through the mouth.

This case demonstrates the beneficial effects of a natural therapy diet on a chronic inflammatory condition of the skin. By restricting the intake of carbohydrates and fats, the secretion of the fatty substance (sebum) is reduced and the skin thus becomes less greasy and less inflamed. It should be noted that the patient wholly recovered.

Case 11: Multiple sclerosis

A woman aged 30 developed typical signs of multiple sclerosis: transient difficulty of vision, tenderness, numbness, stiffness and heaviness of her legs with progressive weakness which made walking difficult. A specialist was consulted who found the power of her right leg had been diminished by 80 to 90 per cent, of her left leg by 50 per cent. Within a few days, the power in the left leg decreased further.

She consulted a natural therapist who prescribed a drastic change from her conventional diet. He followed the instructions given by the German physician, Dr Evers, who had found that sprouting wheat and rye benefited patients suffering from multiple sclerosis. The value of sprouting grains has already been stressed. As we saw, they are extremely rich in various vitamins and they contain first-class proteins. The patient followed the instructions for sprouting and keeping the grains clean (see pages 65-6). In addition she was allowed every day two pints of milk, one raw egg and raw grated root vegetables. She also received a homoeopathic remedy, prepared from an Indian Vetch.

There was an immediate improvement: the strength of her legs increased and the spasm lessened. Hot compresses were applied to relax the stiff muscles. Within two months, the patient had a fair degree of mobility and was able to co-ordinate her movements. As her gait was still uncertain, however, she was put in touch with a teacher of the Matthias Alexander system (see page 102). Already, in the first lesson, the patient's sense of balance was restored. She continued the exercises for a while and derived further benefit from them.

After two months of treatment, her diet was increased: she added wholemeal bread and a full salad (including leaf vegetables), but she kept off tea and coffee for a whole year, and off alcohol for two years.

After four months on the regime she was practically well. There was only some slight unsteadiness of her hands, and she felt ready to look for a job again. After a further four months, she complained of tiredness and jerking of one leg. Two homoeopathic medicines, prepared from lead and the poison nut (*nux vomica*), brought relief. She was also given breathing exercises which she continued. Her last consultation was fifteen months from the beginning of the treatment. Apart from some difficulty in falling asleep and slight twitching of her legs, she had no complaints. She received a high potency of the poison hemlock.

She got married and had two children. Twenty years after she had started the treatment, she reported that she was still following a lacto-vegetarian diet. She always took wholemeal bread. Her health was excellent and she had not suffered any recurrence of her symptoms. At the age of 50 she took up tennis!

Multiple sclerosis is a disease which fluctuates. In this case the recovery followed immediately upon the commencement of a comprehensive treatment on natural lines, including diet, water treatment, massage, exercises and homoeopathic medicine. The excellent permanent cure must be attributed to natural therapy which the patient continued, having adopted its principles as a way of living.

Case 12: Acute sinusitis
A woman aged 43 consulted a natural therapist on account of an attack of acute nasal sinusitis. She had been ill for three days, and an antibiotic had given little relief. She had a slight temperature, her nose felt stuffy, and she had a severe headache.

She was put on a strict diet consisting of fruit, yoghurt, raw salad and cottage cheese. She received an acupuncture treatment which immediately freed her nasal passage and relieved her headache. In addition she was given a homoeopathic medicine, made from slaked lime. She recovered, but was advised to continue with the strict diet for two weeks, and then to add some cooked food.

This case has been quoted to illustrate the handling of an acute illness by natural therapy. If the fever is high, fasting on water and fruit juices is prescribed, and cold compresses around the waist are applied in order to encourage the elimination of toxins through the skin. Appropriate homoeopathic medicines are also used. In less acute cases, such as this one, raw vegetables and fruit with yoghurt constitute a suitable diet.

Notes

Introduction: Nature's balance

1 John Black, *The Dominion of Man: the Search for Ecological Responsibility*, Edinburgh, Edinburgh University Press, 1970, p. 44.

2 Barbara Ward, and René Dubos, *Only One Earth: the Care and Maintenance of a Small Planet*, London, André Deutsch, 1972, p. 115.

3 Harry A. Walters, *Ecology, Food and Civilization*, London, Charles Knight & Co., 1973, p. 192.

4 Anthony Tucker, 'The sludge that threatens the foundation of Britain's farming heritage', *Guardian*, 20 September 1984, p. 13.

5 A.H. Walters, J.R. Fletcher and S.J. Law, 'Nitrate in vegetables: estimation by HPLC', *Nutrition and Health*, A.B. Academic Publishers, vol. 4, no. 3, 1986, p. 148.

6 A. Howard, *An Agricultural Testament*, London, Oxford University Press, 1943 (Special edn, Rodale Press, 1972).

7 T. Vogt, 'Study of possible relation between aluminium in drinking water and dementia', Oslo, Central Bureau of Statistics in Norway, 1986.

8 US Environmental Protection Agency, 'Air Quality for Ozone and other Photochemical Oxidants', Washington, 1986.

9 D. Bellinger *et al.*, 'Low-level lead exposures and early development in socioeconomically disadvantaged children' (abstract), Edinburgh Workshop, quoted in Adam Markham, *The Perils of Vehicle Emissions*, London, Friends of the Earth, July 1987, p. 22.

10 R. Russell-Jones, 'The health effect of vehicle emissions', London, Friends of the Earth, quoted in Markham, op. cit., p. 22.

11 N. Kaoch and M. Schneiderman, *Explaining the Urban Factor in Lung Cancer Mortality: Report to the Natural Resources Defence Council*, Washington, quoted in Markham op. cit., p. 23.

12 C. Holman, *Air Pollution from Diesel Vehicles*, London, Friends of the Earth, July 1987, p. 23.

13 A. Markham, *The Aerosol Connection*, quoted in Markham, op. cit., p. 22.

14 *Friends of the Earth's Second Incident Report, Chemical Trespass: Whose Turn Next?* Pesticides Campaign, London, Friends of the Earth, October 1987, p. 7.

15 A. Harry Walters, op. cit., pp. 172, 173.

16 ibid., p. 177.

Chapter 1: Whom can you trust with your health?

1 David Thomas Reilly, 'Young doctors' views on alternative medicine', *British Medical Journal*, 30 July 1983.

2 Richard Taylor, *Medicine out of Control, The Anatomy of a Malignant Technology*, Melbourne, Sun Books, 1979, p. 1.

3 ibid., pp. 7,8.

4 ibid., p. 23.

5 Sir Macfarlane Burnet, *Genes, Dreams and Realities*, Aylesbury, Medical and Technical Publishing Co., 1971, p. 218.

6 Leslie Kenton, 'Raw energy - nutrition of the future?', *Nutrition and Health*, A.B. Academic Publishers, vol. 4, no. 1, 1985, pp. 38,40.

7 Bernard Dixon, *Beyond the Magic Bullet*, London, George Allen & Unwin, 1978, pp. 222,223.

8 T. Smith, 'Alternative medicine', *British Medical Journal*, 30 July 1983, pp. 307,308; leading article, 'Alternative medicine is no alternative', *Lancet*, 1 October 1983, p. 773; C. Glymour and D. Stalker, 'Engineers, cranks, physicians, magicians', *New England Journal of Medicine*, 21 April 1983, pp. 960-3.

9 Smith, op. cit., p. 307.

10 Glymour and Stalker, op. cit., p. 963.

11 Leading article, *Lancet*, p. 773.

12 I. Smith, letter to the *Lancet*, 22 October 1983, p. 972.

13 Thomas Dummer, 'Why osteopathy is an independent system of medicine', *Journal of Alternative Medicine*, September 1983, p. 8.

Chapter 2: Science in relation to your body

1 R.G. Collingwood, *Speculum Mentis or The Map of Knowledge*, Oxford, Clarendon Press, 1924, p. 166.

2 D.R. Laurence and P.N. Bennett, *Clinical Pharmacology*, Edinburgh, London and New York, Churchill Livingstone, 1980, p. 10.

3 Sir Derrick Dunlop, 'Use and abuse of drugs', *British Medical Journal*, 21 August 1965.

4 See Richard Taylor, *Medicine Out of Control. The Anatomy of a Malignant Technology*, Melbourne, Sun Books, 1979.

5 J.H. Woodger, *Biological Principles, A Critical Study*, London, Kegan Paul, Trench, Trubner & Co., 1929, pp. 242,310.

Chapter 3: Wholeness in relation to your body

1 I. Kant, *Critique of Teleological Judgement* [[1790]], Oxford, Clarendon Press, 1928, p. 34.

2 G.H. Bell, J.N. Davidson and H. Scarborough, *Textbook of Physiology and Biochemistry*, 7th edn, Edinburgh and London, E.S. Livingstone, 1968, p. 655.

3   'Diet and bowel cancer', *British Medical Journal*, 31 May 1980.
4   A. Wright and Gibney Burstyn, 'Dietary fibre and blood pressure', *British Medical Journal*, 15 December 1979.
5   R. Bedford, *The Deadly Cloud, A Health Education Council Publication on Smoking and How to Give it Up*, 1971, pp. 8,3.
6   'The avoidable holocaust. Past irresponsibility', leading article *British Medical Journal*, 5 April 1980.
7   'Views', *British Medical Journal*, 7 March 1981.
8   O. Zetterström, K Osterman, L. Machado and S.G.O. Johansson, 'Another smoking hazard: raised serum IgE concentration and increased risk of occupational allergy', *British Medical Journal*, 7 November 1981.
9   'Action on alcohol is born, *British Medical Journal*, 17 September 1983.
10 P. Small, T. Stockwell and R. Hodgson 'Alcohol dependence and phobic anxiety states: a prevalence study', *British Journal of Psychiatry*, 144, January 1984, p. 53.
11 'Views', *British Medical Journal*, 30 November 1985.
12 R. Bridgewater *et al.* 'Alcohol consumption and dependence in elderly patients in an urban community', *British Medical Journal*, 10 October 1987.
13 D.R. Laurence and P.N. Bennett, *Clinical Pharmacology*, Edinburgh and London, Churchill Livingstone, 1980, pp. 538,539.
14. C.S. Farcas, 'Tea and iron-deficiency anaemia', letter, *British Medical Journal*, 23 February 1980.
15 J.F. Greden, 'Anxiety or caffeinism? A diagnostic dilemma', *American Journal of Psychiatry*, 10 October 1974.
16 G.J. Naylor, L. Grant and C. Smith, 'The effects of caffeine on psychological functioning', *Nutrition and Health*, A.B. Academic Publishers, vol. 4, no. 1, 1985, pp. 33,34.
17 'Views', *British Medical Journal*, 22 March 1986, p. 831, quoted from *American Journal of Obstetrics and Gynecology*, 154, 1986, pp. 14-20.
18 'The avoidable holocaust. Past irresponsibility', leading article, *British Medical Journal*, 5 April 1980.
19 Laurence and Bennett op. cit., p. 538.
20 'Does the pill reduce the risk of some cancers?' quotation of opinion of Sir Charles Dodds, voiced in 1971, *New Health*, London, Haymarket Publications, February 1984, p. 48.

Chapter 4: Natural treatment - the test for holism

1   C. Glymour, and D. Stalker, 'Engineers, cranks, physicians, magicians, *New England Journal of Medicine*, 21 April 1983, p. 963.
2   ibid., p. 962.
3   Ross Trattler, *Better Health through Natural Healing. How to Get Well*

without Drugs or Surgery, Wellingborough, Thorsons Publishing Group, 1987, p. 6.

4   ibid.
5   ibid., pp. 7-9.
6   ibid., p. 63.
7   ibid.
8   ibid., p. 116.
9   ibid., p. 62.
10 E. Atkins, 'Fever - new perspectives on an old phenomenon', *New England Journal of Medicine,* vol. 308, no. 16, 21 April 1983, pp. 958-9.
11 J.S. Patton, letter, 'Treatment of fever', *New England Journal of Medicine,* vol. 309, no. 15, 1983, p. 925.
12 E. Atkins, letter, in ibid., p. 925.

Chapter 5: Food and your health

1   Notice, *British Medical Journal,* 7 September 1985.
2   'Tests raise doubt over food additive: urgent tests on E number', *Health Express,* October 1987, p. 1.
3   C. Curtis Shears, *Nutritional Science and Health Education* published by the author, 1974, p. 94.
4   Weston A. Price, *Nutrition and Physical Degeneration. A Comparison of Primitive and Modern Diets and their Effects,* private publication, 1020 Campus Ave, Redlands, California, 1939.
5   James Lambert Mount, *The Food and Health of Western Man,* London & Tonbridge, Charles Knight & Company,   1975, p. 164.
6   See page 2.
7   A.H. Walters, J.R. Fletcher, and S.J. Law, 'Nitrate in vegetables: estimation by HPLC', *Nutrition and Health.* A.B. Academic Publishers, vol. 4, no. 3, 1986, p. 149.
8   Ross Hume Hall, *Food for Nought. The Decline in Nutrition,* New York, Evanston, San Francisco, London, Harper & Row, 1974, p. 52.
9   ibid., Preface, ix.
10 Committee on Diet, Nutrition, and Cancer. Assembly of Life Sciences, National Research Council, *Diet, Nutrition, and Cancer,* National Academic Press, Washington DC, 1982.
11 ibid., chpt. 5 p. 4.
12 ibid., chpt. 5 pp. 6,7.
13 *Journal of the National Cancer Institute,* 77:605-12, quoted in Views, *British Medical Journal* 22 November 1986.
14 *Diet, Nutrition, and Cancer,* chpt. 6 p. 1.
15 See page 29.
16 *Diet, Nutrition, and Cancer,* chpt. 9 p. 7.
17 ibid., chpt. 10 p. 25.

18   *Diet, Nutrition and Cancer,* chpt. 12 p. 20.
19   ibid. chpt. 15 p. 1.
20   ibid. chpt. 15 p. 9.
21   T.L. Cleave and G.D. Campbell, 'Research review: the saccharine disease', *Medical News,* 16 June 1967.
22   T.L. Cleave and G.D. Campbell, *Diabetes, Coronary Thrombosis and the Saccharine Disease,* Bristol, John Wright & Sons, 1966, p.31.
23   T.L. Cleave and G.D. Campbell *Medical News,* 16 June 1967.
24   A. Wright, P.G. Burstyn and M.J. Gibney, 'Dietary fibre and blood pressure', *British Medical Journal,* 15 December 1979.
25   R.C. Trowell and D.P. Burkitt, 'Fibre and disease', *On Call,* 27 October 1977, pp. 13,14.
26   The Second Fisons Food Allergy Workshop, Medical Education Services Ltd, Symposium Highlights, 1983, p. 3.
27   J. Runcie and T.E. Hildich, 'Energy provision, tissue utilisation and weight loss in prolonged starvation', *British Medical Journal,* 18 May 1974.
28   E.J. Drenick *et al.,* 'Prolonged starvation as treatment for severe obesity', *Journal of the American Medical Association,* vol. 187:100-5, 1964, summarized as 'Total starvation in weight reduction' in *Modern Medicine of Great Britain,* April 1965.
29   H.M. Shelton, *Fasting Can Save Your Life,* Chicago, Natural Hygiene Press, 1964, p.15.
30   E. Heun, 'Regeneration durch Hungern', Fasten und Rohsäfte', *Hippokrates,* Heft 15, Stuttgart, 1960.
31   C. Curtis Shears, op. cit., p.76.
32   D.C. Hare, 'A therapeutic trial of a raw vegetable diet in chronic rheumatic conditions', *Proceedings of the Royal Society of Medicine,* vol. 30, no. 1, 1936.
33   D.C. Hare and E.C. Pillman-Williams, 'Vitamin C output in diet treatment of rheumatoid arthritis', *Lancet,* vol. 1, no. 20, 1938.
34   L.A. Carlson and S.O. Froberg, 'Blood liquid and glucose levels during a ten-day period of low-calorific intake and exercise in man' *Metabolism,* vol. 16, no. 624, 1967.
35   Massamori Kuratsune, 'Experiment on low nourishment with raw vegetables', Kyushu Memoirs of Medical Sciences, 2 June 1951.
36   R.J.L. Allen, M. Brook and S.R. Broadbent, 'The variability of Vitamin C in our diet', *British Journal of Nutrition,* vol. 22, no. 555, 1968.
37   R.J.W. Burrell, W.A. Roach and A. Shadwell, 'Esophageal cancer in the Bantu of the Transkei associated with mineral deficiency in garden plants', *Journal of the National Cancer Institute,* vol. 36, no. 201, 1966.
38   J.J. Segall, 'Cardiovascular disease and peptic ulcer', letter in *British Medical Journal,* 18 January 1975.

39 D.F. Davies *et al.*, 'Cow's milk antibodies and coronary heart disease', letter, *Lancet*, 31 May 1980, pp. 1190-1191.

40 B. Jacobson, 'Stones of affluence', *World Medicine*, 27 August 1975.

41 T.H. Crouch, 'Dietary immunology: an hypothesis', *New Zealand Medical Journal*, vol. 76, no. 486, 1972, pp. 372-3.

42 T.L. Cleave and G.D. Campbell, *Diabetes, Coronary Thrombosis and the Saccharine Disease*, Bristol, John Wright & Sons, 1966.

43 C. Curtis Shears, op. cit., p.150.

44 ibid., pp. 129, 130.

45 'Position paper on the vegetarian approach to eating', *Journal of the American Dietetic Association*, vol. 77, no. 1, 1980, pp. 1161-9.

46 Barrie M. Margetts, 'Vegetarian diet in mild hypertension. A random mixed controlled trial', *British Medical Journal*, 6 December 1986; and E. Ernst *et al.*, 'Vegetarian diet in mild hypertension' *British Medical Journal* 17 January 1987, p. 180.

47 A. Long, 'The well-nourished vegetarian', *New Scientist*, 5 February 1981.

48 S.S. Gear *et al.*, 'Symptomless diverticular disease and intake of dietary fibre', *Lancet*, 10 March 1979, pp. 511-13.

49 J.R. Thornton *et al.*, 'Diet in Crohn's disease: Characteristics of the pre-illness diet', *British Medical Journal* 29 September 1979.

50 P.S. Davies and J. Rhodes, 'Maintenance of a remission in ulcerative colitis with sulphasalazine or a high fibre diet: a clinical trial', *British Medical Journal*, 10 June 1987.

51 Gerald J. Friedman, 'Diet in treatment of diabetes mellitus', in *Modern Nutrition in Health and Disease*, ed R.S. Goodhart and M.E. Shils, 6th edn, London, Henry Kimpton, 1980.

52 A. Long, 'The well-nourished vegetarian', *New Scientist*, 5 February 1981.

53 'Vegetarianism for the kidneys. A VSUK-supported project finds that diets high in vegetable protein have beneficial effects on the kidneys', Research Section, Dr Alan Long, *The Vegetarian*, September/October 1987, p. 33.

54 Lowell S. Selling and Mary Anna Ferraro, *The Psychology of Diet and Nutrition*, London, Bodley Head, 1947, p.12.

55 J. Trevor Silverstone, 'Psychological and social aspects of obesity', *British Journal of Hospital Medicine*, July 1973.

56 Quoted from L.J. Mount, *The Food and Health of Western Man*, London, Charles Knight, 1975, p. 237.

Chapter 6: Health and your bowel

1   See pages 47-8.

2   Committee on Diet, Nutrition, and Cancer. Assembly of Life Sciences, National Research Council, *Diet, Nutrition, and Cancer*, National

Academic Press, Washington DC, 1982, chpt. 5 p. 9.

3   ibid., chpt. 5 pp. 17,18,19.

4   V. Aries *et al.*, 'Bacteria and the aetiology of cancer of the large bowel', *Gut,* 10, 1969, pp. 334-5.

5   For a summary of the role played by intestinal flora see, for instance, Gary L. Simon and Sherwood L. Gorbach, 'The human intestinal microflora', *Digestive Diseases and Sciences,* vol. 31, no. 9, Supplement, 1986, pp. 1475-1625.

6   Quoted from E.D. Wittkower, *Einfluss der Gemütsbewegungen auf den Körper,* second edition, Wien, Leipzig, Sensen Verlag, 1937, pp. 101,102.

7   H.M. Shelton, *Fasting Can Save Your Life,* Chicago, Natural Hygiene Press, 1964, p. 68

Chapter 7: The breath of life

1   Diana Gaskell, 'Domiciliary physiotherapy in the treatment of chronic bronchitis and emphysema', *Update,* May 1970, pp. 587-8.

2   ibid., p. 588.

Chapter 8: Natural stimulation and your skin

1   E.F. St John Lyburn, 'Nine clinical achievements of therapeutic sweating', *Hospital Times,* 6 October 1970.

2   W. Müller-Limmroth and A. Ruffmann, 'Experimentelle Untersuchungen über die physiologischen Sauna-Wirkungen auf den gesunden Menschen', *Hippokrates,* Heft 23, Stuttgart, 15 December 1962.

3   H. Krauss, 'Physikalisch-diätetische Therapie der entzündlichen Rheumakrankheiten', *Hippokrates,* Heft 5, Stuttgart, 1961.

4   'Sauna baths prove to be harmful' *Medical News-Tribune,* vol. 2, no. 43, 23 October 1970.

5   Clifford Hawkins, 'The sauna: killer or healer?', *British Medical Journal,* 24 October 1987, pp. 1015,1016.

6   ibid.

7   A. Hoff, 'Allgemeines und Spezielles aus der Naturheilkunde', *Hippokrates,* Stuttgart, 31 August 1947.

8   Father Kneipp, *My Water Cure,* Edinburgh, William Blackwood & Sons, 1891.

9   K. Franke, 'Die Bedeutung der kleinen Hydrotherapie (nach Kneipp) fur die Prävention und Rehabilitation von Arthritis und Kollagen-Krankheiten am Gefässsystem' *Hippokrates,* Heft 3, Stuttgart, 1961.

10 F. Velse, 'Physikalische und diätetische Behandlung des Bluthochdrucks', *Archiv für Physikalische Therapie,* Heft 4, 1966.

11 For a summary of the effects of the ground and air on the skin, see Gerhard Kunze, *Physiatrie, Naturrztliche Rundschau,* August 1932.

12 'Sun, wind and the skin', *British Medical Journal*, 13 July 1974.
13 A. Rollier, *Heliotherapy*, Oxford Medical Publications, London, Henry Frowde and Hodder & Stoughton, 1923.
14 ibid.
15 A. Rollier, *The International Factory Clinic for the Treatment by Sun and Work of Indigent Cases of 'Surgical' Tuberculosis*, Paris, Librarie Payot et Cie, 1929.
16 Edward Mayer, *Radiation and Climatic Therapy of Chronic Pulmonary Diseases with Special Reference to Natural and Artificial Heliotherapy, X-Ray and Climatic Therapy of Chronic Pulmonary Diseases and All Forms of Tuberculosis*, Baltimore, The Williams & Wilkins Co., 1944.

Chapter 9: Posture, exercise and relaxation
1 Charles A. Neill, *Poise and Relaxation*, A Family Doctor Publication, London (now out of print).
2 ibid.
3 Kenneth Crutchfield, 'Exercise' in Cooper Ernest (ed.) *Health in the Home: The Food Reform and Nature Cure Manual*, London Health Centre Ltd. and National Association of Health Stores, London, 1948.
4 Kenneth H. Cooper, *The New Aerobics*, New York, Bantam Books, 1970.
5 ibid.
6 Thomas Semple, 'Exercise in prevention of coronary heart disease', *Health Magazine, vol. 2, no. 1, Spring 1974.*
7 J.C. Houston, C.L. Joiner and J.R. Trounce, *A Short Textbook of Medicine*, London, English Universities Press Ltd, 1968, p.386.
8 W. Lübken, 'Bewegung und Hydrotherapie in der Diabetesbehandlung' *Hippokrates*, Heft 8, Stuttgart, 1961.
9 Johannes H. Schultz and Wolfgang Luthe, *Autogenic Training, a Psychophysiologic Approach in Psychotherapy*, New York, Grune & Stratton, 1959.

Chapter 10: Allies to natural therapy
1 See E.K. Ledermann, 'Homoeopathy and natural therapeutics', *The British Homoeopathic Journal*, vol. XXXV, no. 1, May 1945; and E.K. Ledermann, 'The philosophical and scientific basis of alopathic and homoeopathic medicine', *The British Homoeopathic Journal*, vol. XXXIV, nos 2,3, September 1944.
2 See E.K. Ledermann, 'Implications of Hahnemannian homoeopathy', *The British Homoeopathic Journal*, vol. XLVI, no. 4, October 1957.
3 See for example the animal experiments which demonstrate such connections, quoted in Felix Mann, *Acupuncture: The Ancient Chinese Art of Healing*, London, William Heinemann Medical Books, 1971; and Mann, *Scientific Aspects of Acupuncture*, London, William Heineman Medical Books, 1983.

4   See for instance, D.N. Golding, 'Indications for acupuncture in back pain', *Acupuncture in Medicine, Journal of the British Acupuncture Society*, vol. IV, no. 2, November/December 1987.

5   See for instance, Erich H Stiefvater, *What is Acupuncture? How does it work?* second edition, Health Science Press, 1971.

6   Paul Renard, 'Pathologie-Psychologie et Acupuncture', second instalment, *Revue Trimestrielle de l'Organisation pour l'Etude et le Dévelopement de l'Acupuncture*, 11e année, No 41, July, August, September 1974.

7   Otto Bergsmann, *Objektivierung der Akupunktur als Problem der Regulationsphysiologie*, Heidelberg, Verlag Haug, 1974.

8   Marshall Hoag, Wilbur V. Cole and Spencer G. Bradford, *Osteopathic Medicine*, New York, Blakiston Division/McGraw-Hill, 1969.

9   ibid. For a recent formulation see, for instance, Peter Hawkins, *Osteopathy*, published by author, London, 1986.

10   Anthea Courtenay, *Chiropractic for Everyone*, Harmondsworth, Penguin Books, 1987.

11   Elisabeth Dicke, *Meine Bindegewebsmassage*, Hippokrates-Verlag, 2nd edition, 1954, English version: Maria Ebner, *Connective Tissue Massage: Theory and Therapeutic Applications*, Edinburgh and London, E.& S. Livingstone, 1962.

Name Index

Note: References to names that have been directly mentioned in the text have been **emboldened**, the others have been quoted or referred to without being specifically named in the text.

Subject Index

0700073150

A/C - 0602574-05/1